The Art of
Q *the*
uickie

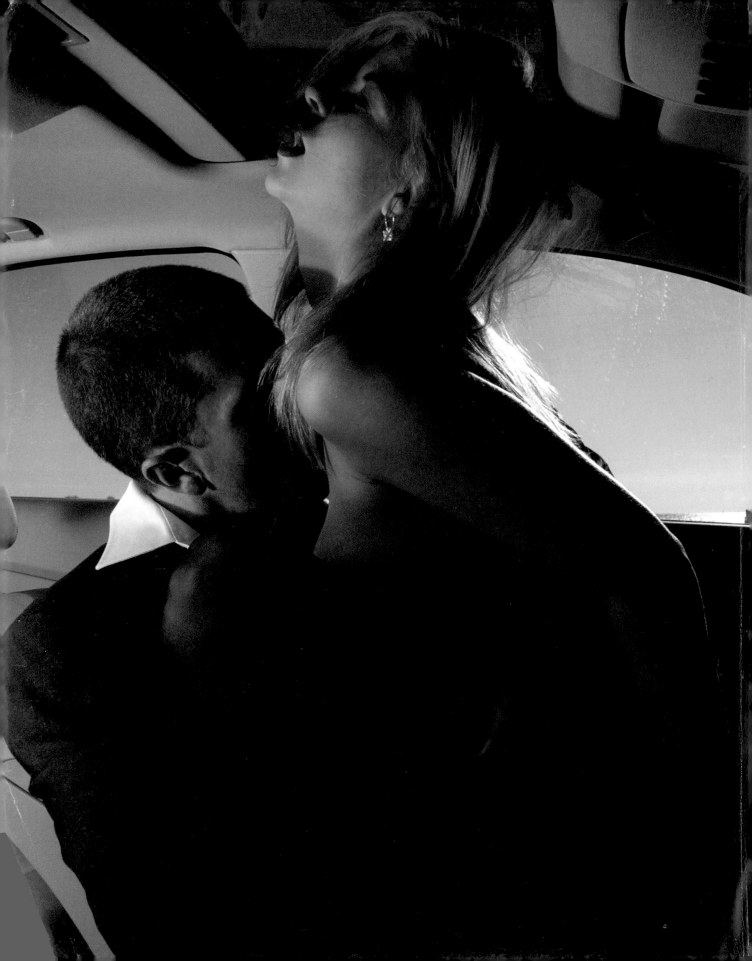

The Art of
the
Quickie

Fast Sex | Fast Orgasm | Anytime, Anywhere

Joel D. Block, Ph.D.

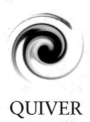

QUIVER

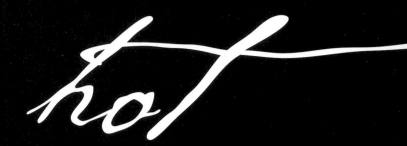

Text © 2006 Pop Psych Literary, Inc.

Photography © 2006 Rockport Publishers

First published in the USA in 2006 by
Quiver, a member of
Quayside Publishing Group
33 Commercial Street
Gloucester, MA 01930

10 09 08 07 06   1 2 3 4 5

ISBN-13: 978-1-59233-240-3
ISBN-10: 1-59233-240-4

Library of Congress Cataloging-in-Publication Data
Block, Joel D.
  The art of the quickie : fast sex/fast orgasm/anytime, anywhere / Joel D. Block.
    p. cm.
  ISBN-13: 978-1-59233-240-3
  ISBN-10: 1-59233-240-4
  1. Sex instruction. 2. Orgasm. I. Title.
  HQ31.B565 2006
  613.9'6--dc22

                                             2006019573

Cover and book design by Carol Holtz Design
Photography by Allan Penn

INTRODUCTION

WELCOME TO FAST CITY

Chemistry is at peak levels and every look exchanged is full of lust and promise. You leap on each other before you leave the house in the morning and flash back to your lovemaking throughout the day.

Greeting each other in the evening is anticipated with the kind of excitement people reserve for special occasions. You feel as if you are continually dressing because you're taking your clothes off so often, but you don't mind the extra effort one bit...

Sound familiar? Probably not. If anything, this is likely a distant memory of those first months of your relationship. Don't weep; you've picked up an exciting plan for rekindling that passion.

I specialize in working with couples—treating them, writing about them, giving them presentations, and answering their emails. The subject invariably turns to sex and the complaints are often the same: They have no time for sex. They miss having sex. They want to know how to improve their sex lives. Sex has been missing from their relationship and they are looking for ways to bring sexual passion back. They want ideas of how to find time for sex.

Here are some of the comments I've heard concerning this hot topic:

"By the time I get to bed, all I'm thinking about is sleep! The other day it dawned on me that I couldn't remember the last time we had sex."

"I know that everyone says to just make a date night, but when? It's not as easy as it seems."

"Sometimes it seems that my husband and I are more like roomies or friends than married, because we spend so much time on other things, not the passion we had early on."

"We have sex, now and then, but it feels like something on the 'to do' list. Pick up milk. Drop Darren off at karate. Mail the bills. Have sex. Sex isn't even first on the list!"

"When I think of finding the time or energy for sex I get discouraged. Frankly, there's not enough in it for me to make the effort. That's a long way from the early days when we couldn't keep our hands off each other!"

"After we have sex I always think, What happened to the excitement we used to have? The Wow! factor. Something that would lead me to say to myself, 'that's great, let's do it more often.' After working all day, making dinner, doing chores, giving the kids some attention and putting them to bed, I need an incentive."

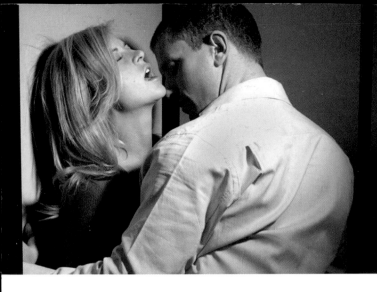

Not a pretty picture. Many of today's couples think of lovemaking as something that has to be worked up to gradually and with delicacy. It's assumed that a large block of time has to be put aside for the encounter, and they can't manage to find it. Although this kind of lovemaking can certainly be a luxurious part of an intimate relationship, so too are those unplanned moments when you just feel like having sex with no preparation at all.

Asking you if you would like a richer, fuller, more intensely pleasurable and rewarding sex life is like asking if you would object to inheriting a few million dollars, no strings attached and taxes already paid. Almost everyone wants better sex.

Even if it's good we want it better. Sexual passion has the power to lift our spirits unlike any other feeling, just as sexual frustration can dampen our spirits unlike any other experience.

So, what makes more sense when it comes to our sex lives—the infrequent feast or the more frequent delicious snack that creates a hunger for more? What do the experts suggest? Put more romance in your life! A cottage industry has sprung up to address what is perceived to be the problem: no time, no energy, and no opportunity for sex. The experts' advice: schedule, plan, make dates, be more romantic, blah, blah, blah.

Lots of us tried to follow the experts' advice only to end up feeling that we were doing something wrong because it wasn't working. But we're not wrong! The experts have it wrong, and, with full disclosure, I have been among them.

Humans were designed for faster and bolder sex. That's right. Not only faster, but also, at least on occasion, with a bit of daring behavior thrown in. We require novelty. Historically, the animal kingdom didn't waste time. The more time spent on sex, the more vulnerable they were to being consumed. And the consumption being referred to isn't oral sex!

In addition, it is likely that we will be in a relationship longer than our ancestors lived. Sex, after a few hundred repetitions of ten minutes of foreplay followed by two minutes of thrusting in the missionary position, can easily become routine and boring. To take this evolutionary fact into today's world of long hours at the office, endless traffic, and children to care for, it's a wonder we find time for sex at all, especially since it often doesn't deliver when we do. Sure, the five-course gourmet deal is delicious. But sometimes, nothing but a slice of masterfully topped pizza straight from a wood-fired brick oven will do. It's unrealistic to expect to engage in full-on sex all the time, which is why daring quickies are not optional— they're damn necessary.

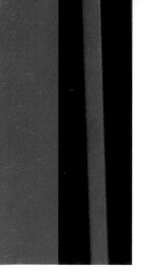

I expect quickies won't be your only way of making love, but, stepping out of your usual routine is an excellent way to keep sexual passion burning.

What do I mean by a quickie?

In case it's not clear, some quickies involve less time than it takes to poach an egg. Some are not speedy and are different, but there is a definite shift in the approach. It's less about romance and more about creating and acting on your lust.

This is totally the opposite of everything you normally hear: set a romantic mood, don't rush things, why rush through something that's so pleasurable? And I say why not! It's all about a shift in attitude.

As we will hear in their own words, lots of women contend that there's something to be said for forgetting the hoopla every once in a while. No hands. No mouths. No talk. Just do it. It's like being told: "I must have you! Now!"

So what if he's shaving and late for work, or you're busy paying the bills? For once, wouldn't it be wild to get swept off your feet (or knock him off his)?

Okay, so you might not have an orgasm because it'll be so quick. That's fine, as long as you enjoy yourself. Sex isn't a competition based on a point system. Variety adds a quality of its own. Besides, I maintain that if you follow the guidelines to come, the chances of having an orgasm are greatly increased. In fact, I'm betting that you'll be more easily orgasmic during a quickie than during routine lovemaking.

Of course, it's a completely different story if all you have are quickies. Or if you never have an orgasm. Or if he always comes too quickly. Because, ultimately, the best sex is an encounter between two people who want to be with each other and have an interest in satisfying each other.

You may be thinking, "Oh, that's great for men, but what about women? Is the quickie fair to them?" For women, the common feeling is that a quickie means the man gets off and she gets left behind—he leaves the party before she even gets there!

It doesn't take much to convince men of the merit of quickies; it's the ultimate guy thing. For women it's a double-edged sword: She may want it but she anticipates she won't likely get much out of it except frustration.

However, I maintain that quickies can be more than fair to women. By adding spontaneity to your sex life—especially when the setting is different and the approach is bold—you will turn up the heat. In fact, once the novelty has waned, spontaneity is required; desire is like a fire with a flame that needs to be stoked. A dose of daring, edgy sex is like oxygen for the flame. But women have a hurdle to overcome: While the penis is stimulated directly during the typical sex encounter, the clitoris is aroused indirectly.

This doesn't mean that women are incapable of reaching orgasm more quickly. In fact, both men and women can usually masturbate themselves to orgasm in less than five minutes—eminent sexuality scientist Alfred Kinsey reported that it takes an average of three minutes for both men and women to come to orgasm when they stimulate themselves.

If you can do it on your own, you can definitely catch the orgasmic express with your partner by using the right techniques. In this book, these techniques will be spelled out in three easy-to-learn steps!

These aren't exotic techniques like something from the Far East that requires years to master. Quite to the contrary, you will learn to become more easily orgasmic in less time than it takes to do the regular food shopping, cooking, laundry, and cleaning— and the sex is going to be much more fun! The premise of this book is simple: **Occasional quickie sex—primal and spontaneous or planned, with mischief and in forbidden locations—where both he AND she get rocked, is just what's needed to bring back the glow of the early days, the days of sex in the hallway.**

We need more than just time to have sex; we need a reason to make it happen. Motivation is key, and novelty pumps motivation. One survey reports that Americans have intercourse an average of sixty-four times a year. That's a bit more than once a week, on average. But it's quality, not quantity that counts. It's not a question of how often, but how pleasurable and how interesting.

Frequent sex is one thing, but memorable sex, the kind that brings an involuntary smile to your face, is what this book is about.

It's been my experience that couples, especially when they've been together a while, often fall victim to the biggest libido killer: monotony. That's when a little creativity, a flexible and open attitude, and a sense of humor can come in handy. But wait a minute. Let's get real. While the great thing about a quickie is that it's a no-frills (or very different frills), anything-goes deal, the reality is that sex rarely happens with complete spontaneity. There is practically always a prelude that leads us to be sexual: something we've seen (that guy in the office with the great buns showing just the right degree of vulnerability), maybe a certain loving touch, or even mid-cycle (about fourteen days after your period) when your body starts screaming Yes! Yes!

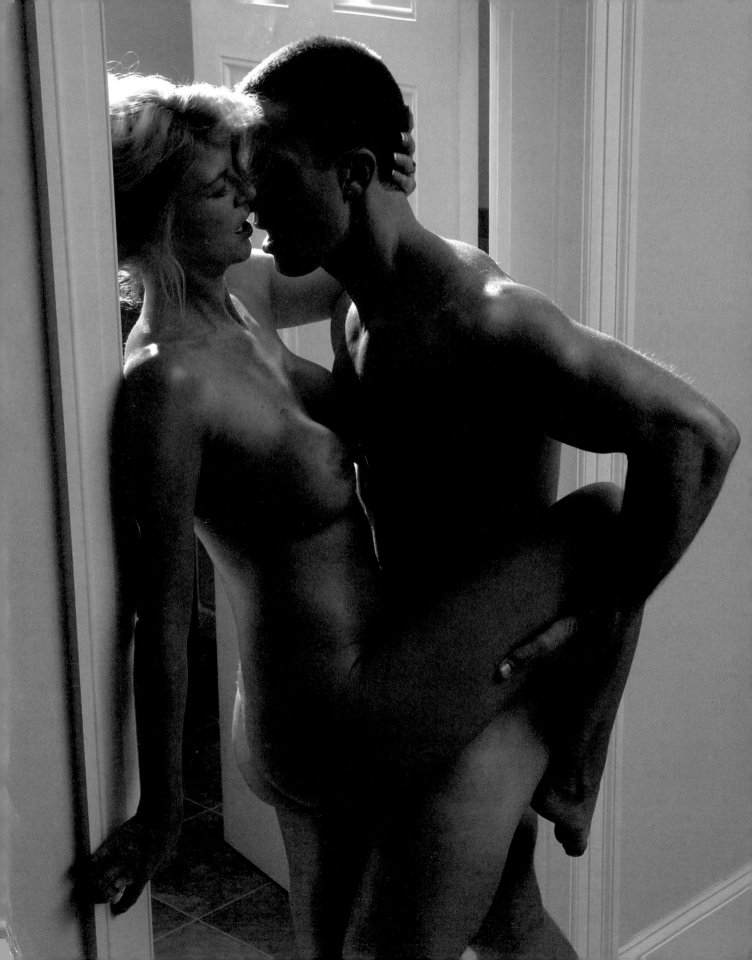

Bottom line: My definition of "quickie" is pretty liberal. This is not by any means your grandmother's quickie, the "wham-bam, thank you, ma'am" duty sex that pleased only the man. These quickies are provocative encounters that may not always be quick but are always different; they break the usual pattern, bringing in elements of daring and the forbidden that are not part of your typical lovemaking. A quickie may not always be speedy, but it should get your blood flowing and incite you into a sexual frenzy.

After all, what's more inspiring than unexpected, animalistic, quick-paced sessions that involve stolen moments in which you both forget about the world for just a little while?

BY BECOMING A QUICKIE *SEXPERT*, YOU WILL:

> heighten your sexual energy.
> practice getting "ready" almost immediately (especially important for women).
> fuel a heightened sexual tension between the two of you.
> substantially increase your level of intimacy.
> help raise testosterone levels in both of you.

An encounter of unbridled passion can bring you more than just intense and passionate pleasure. The urgency can rekindle old, forgotten feelings, and in no time you can be transported back to the early days of your relationship, or even the first hours of your sexual awakening.

You will both get better at this with practice. You will find it highly erotic and very effective for boosting your general energy levels throughout the day; it's better than a double espresso. You'll find yourselves thinking about each other a lot more.

If time permits, the luxury of concentrating on a sensual, lingering build-up to lovemaking is delightful. Yet conditioning yourself for that raw sense of urgency that takes over, the moment when you just can't wait…that's hot!

The point is that a no-holds-barred, rip-off-my-clothes-with-your-teeth-right-here-right-now sex is not only the best way to have more fun in bed, it's also a way to keep a long-term monogamous relationship from feeling like—dare I say it?—a long-term monogamous relationship.

The occasional quickie is to sexual pleasure like spicy marinara sauce added to made-from-scratch pasta: that little something extra that elevates the delicious to the sublime.

QUICKIE

OVERCOME BY THE URGE

A QUICKIE CAN HAPPEN ANYTIME—WHEN YOU WALK IN THE DOOR, WHEN YOU'RE GETTING READY FOR WORK IN THE MORNING, WHEN YOU'RE ON YOUR WAY TO BED—YOU CAN BE OVERCOME BY THE URGE TO HAVE HOT, FAST SEX WHEN YOU LEAST EXPECT IT.

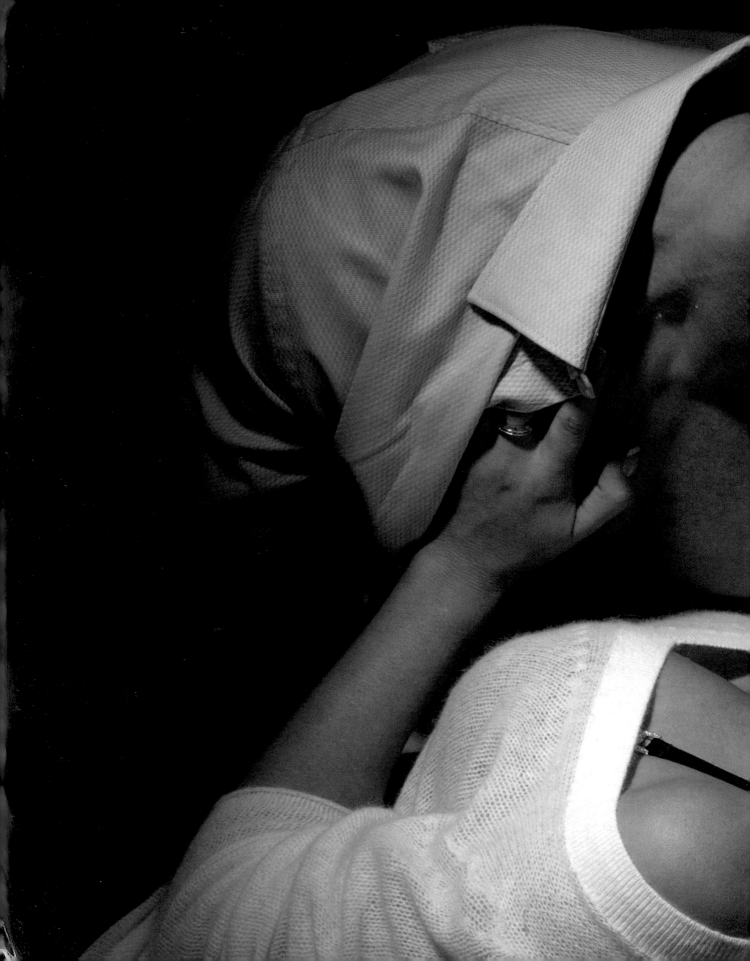

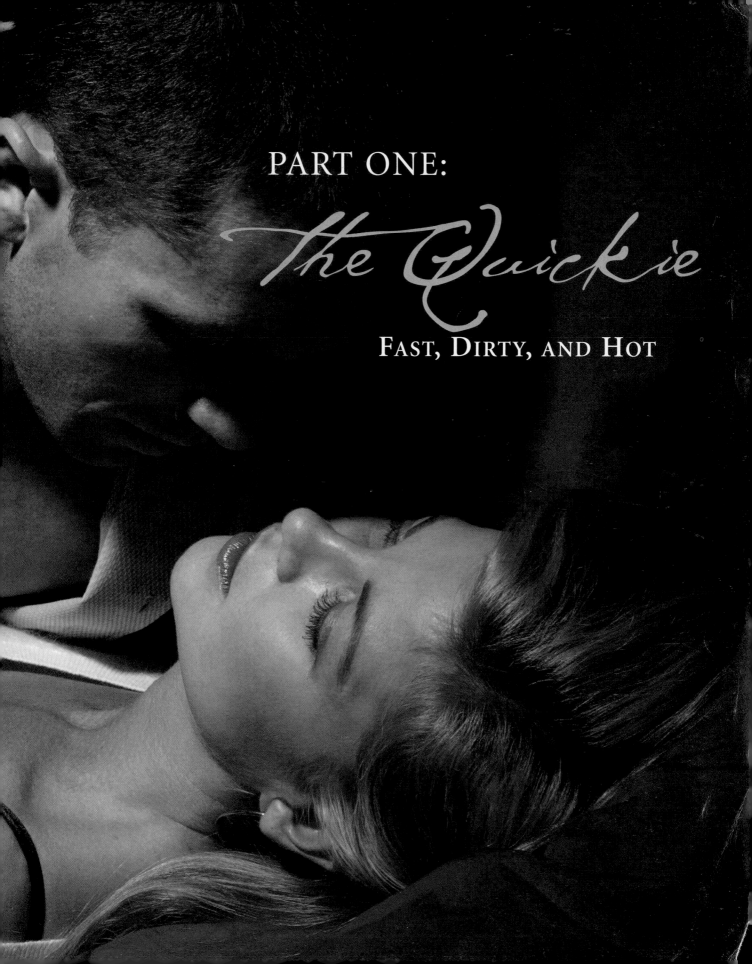

PART ONE:

The Quickie

FAST, DIRTY, AND HOT

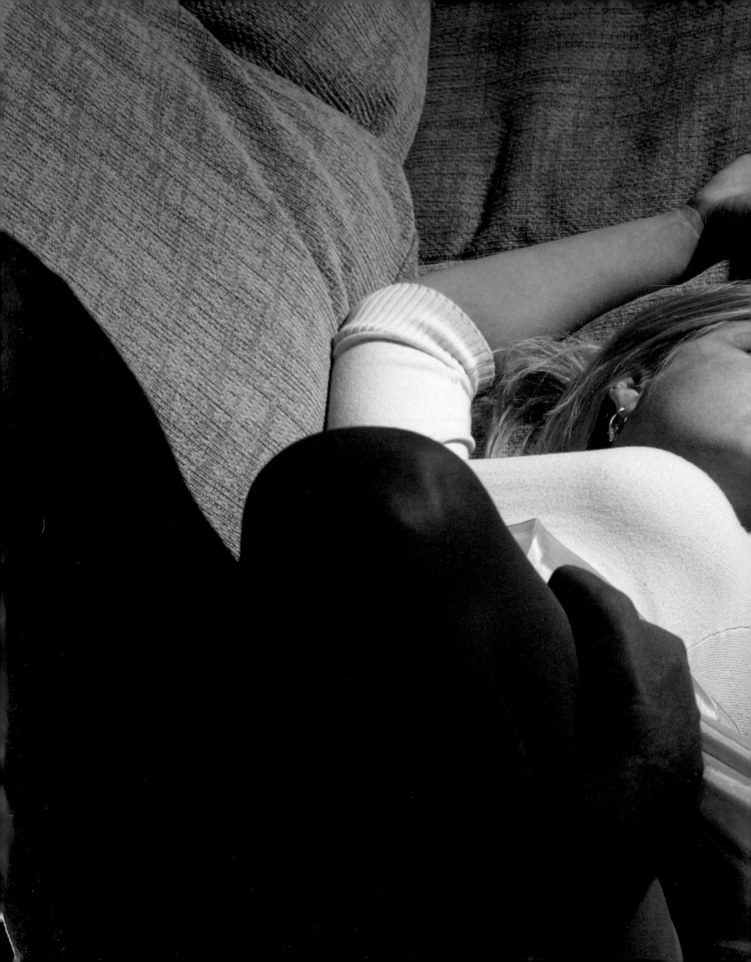

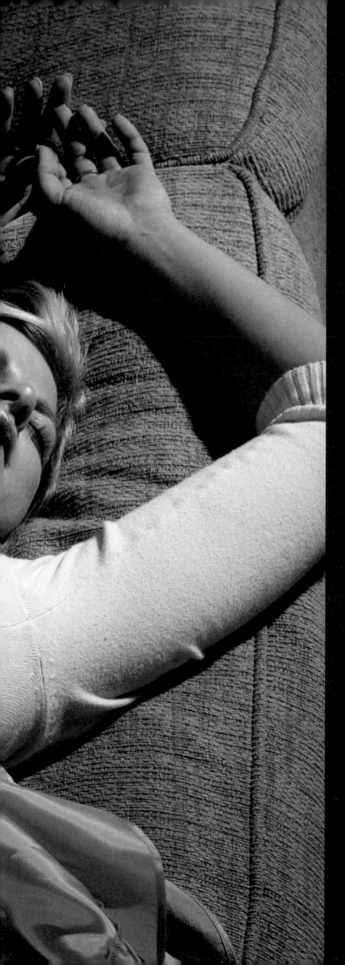

1

What Women Say About Quickies

YOU'RE NOT ALONE!

You may still be skeptical, asking "What's in it for me?" I don't blame you; quickies have a stubborn reputation as being something a woman lends herself to in deference to her man. But boredom and lack of sexual interest among women also has a long and stubborn history.

Unless you keep doing the same thing, history doesn't have to repeat itself. Fess up; you're not always in the mood for a drawn-out marathon of lovin'. Sometimes you're so damned hot you just want to sprint past the tantric sex deal and get down with it. The good news is that all it takes is a little imagination to fire up your sex life. There is nothing so exhilarating as fast, frenzied sex that is impetuous and NOT politically correct—sex that borders on the forbidden and the wild.

Pick and choose from the myriad of suggestions in this book. Put some effort into speeding up your arousal and orgasmic response—I'll show you how—and you'll change your mind about quickies and shatter your boredom. Some women say that quickie sex is better for them than any other approach. Because it often is unplanned, they can simply be taken over by their man's passion and their own.

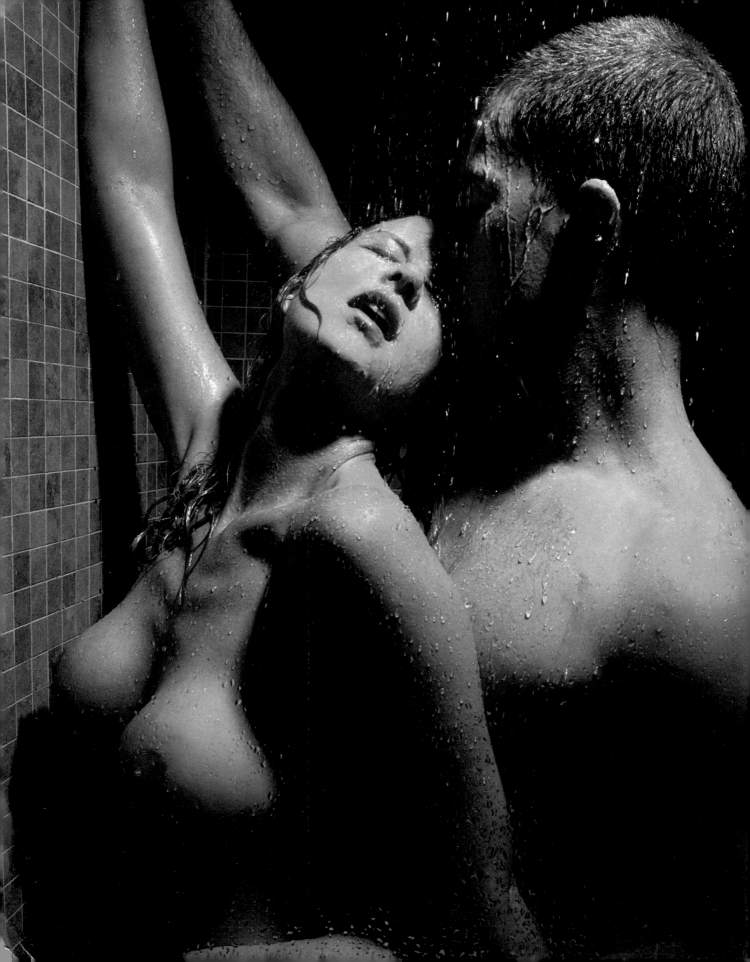

GIRLS BEING NAUGHTY

As one thirty-three-year-old woman told me, "Some of our best memories are quickies, like the time we did it standing up in the dressing room on the Metroliner between D.C. and New York."

Several other women I spoke with weighed in enthusiastically when I asked them about the most adventurous thing they ever did sexually.

A woman in her early twenties had this to say: "On my wedding day, at the reception, I went to a small room to change with my new husband. I was thinking about the wedding, but when he dropped his pants he was fully erect. I got hot just from the way he looked at me and instantly we were getting it on facing each other. All this was happening with people milling around just on the other side of the door. For the rest of the evening, every time we looked at each other surrounded by our guests, we had sly smiles on our faces. If you ask me what I remember most about our wedding, that was it. It's what really made our day special!"

Another woman, also thirty-something, had this to say: "Fast and frantic sex is energizing. About once a week we have a quickie in the shower in the morning before work. It's unscheduled, hot, and we're more charged for lovemaking the next time around."

QUICKIE

STEAMY SHOWER

A STEAMY SHOWER CAN BE THE PERFECT SPOT FOR A SURPRISE QUICKIE. THERE IS A GREAT DEAL OF SEXUAL PLEASURE THAT YOU CAN EXPERIENCE IN WATER—CONSIDERED BY MANY TO BE A SENSUAL APHRODISIAC.

DRESSING ROOM RENDEZVOUS

AN UNUSUAL OR "FORBIDDEN" PLACE OFTEN MAKES THE BEST SETTING FOR A QUICKIE. THIS DRESSING ROOM RENDEZVOUS WOULD MAKE ANY MAN CHANGE HIS MIND ABOUT SHOPPING!

It's a rule of the universe that guys don't like to shop. But as with all rules, there are exceptions, and I'll bet that this thirty-something guy doesn't mind shopping at all.

Here's what his girl told me: "We were shopping for some new clothes for him and he was trying them on in the dressing room. It was late and the store was empty. I stepped into the dressing room with him and rubbed against his underwear. Then our eyes locked. Next thing I knew my arms were above my head and I was being held against the wall. I did my best to keep my moaning as quiet as possible, but I'm afraid the attendant had some suspicion. When we came out of the dressing room he had this look and he glanced at us with knowing eyes. I said something wise-ass to him, I don't remember exactly what, but it was a little flirty. I thought he would come in his pants right then and there."

Have you ever paid a lot of money for an experience and found it disappointing? It's happened to most of us on occasion. It happened to this woman on her fortieth birthday, except she found a unique solution.

"We were at a Broadway play. My boyfriend paid a lot of money for the seats but the play was very slow. I felt bad for him and in the middle of the play I took his hand and led him into the men's room. We went into a stall. Not a word was exchanged between us, just lusty glances at each other. He turned me around and entered me from behind. No one came in, but the thought of it really turned me on. We found our way back to the seats and somehow the play took on new meaning. Afterwards, I asked him if he had found the drama worthwhile. He grinned and told me I deserved the Tony Award for Best Quickie on Broadway."

anywhere

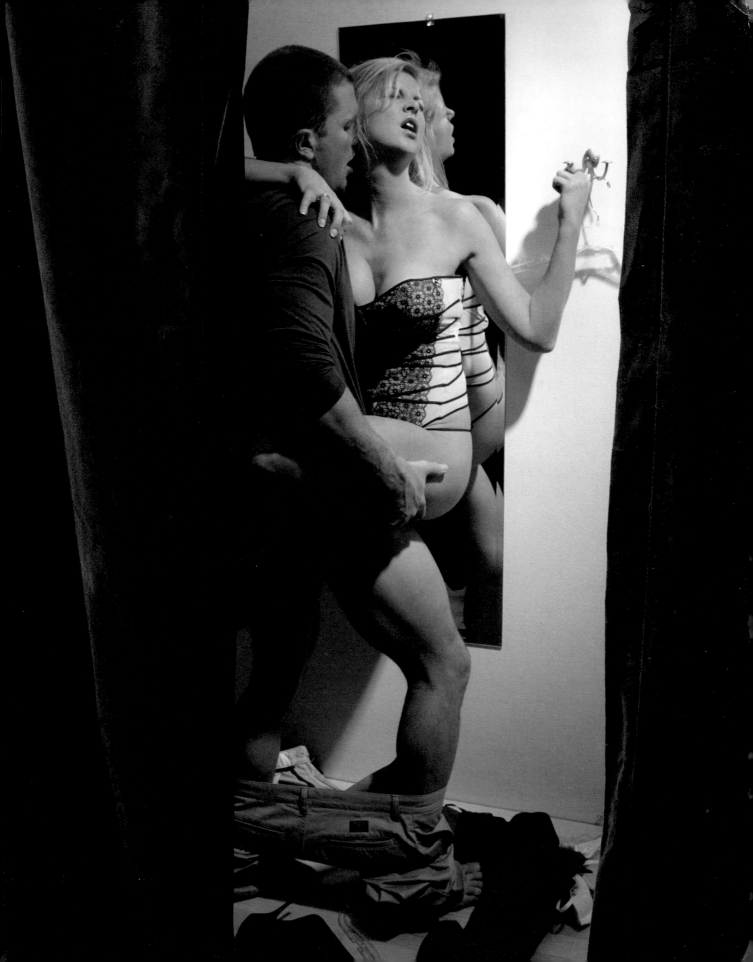

And sometimes, even a vacation can be drab, but add a little drama and it can stir up an award-winning erotic explosion. A recently engaged woman in her mid-thirties can attest to that:

"I was with my fiancé on vacation celebrating our engagement and I purposely wasn't wearing panties. My skirt was loose and he teased me all night. I noticed he was hard all night. We were in the hotel lounge just talking dirty to each other and flirting. Finally, he slipped off his shoe and put his foot between my legs under the table. Less than a minute later I heard myself say, 'Let's go upstairs,' in a surprisingly husky tone. I could feel myself getting very wet. In the elevator I had just pressed the up button when he pulled up my skirt and entered me, face-to-face, very slowly, just barely sliding in and letting me experience the feeling of him inserting his penis in me at a very gentle pace.

"The whole time he was looking directly into my eyes and telling me how wonderful it was feeling to him. I thought I'd lose my mind, it was so hot, just being sexually aroused all evening, thinking and wondering when it would happen. I was so wet! All of him inside of me…then the elevator stopped and the doors opened. We had to compose ourselves. An older couple got on the elevator, looked at us and then smiled at each other. When we got off we continued to make love in the hall and the excitement of getting caught again made me wild. We were just totally aroused for a very long time and couldn't get enough of each other."

QUICKIE

GOING UP!

HAVING A QUICKIE IN AN ELEVATOR IS DARING AND EXCITING! HOWEVER, MAKE SURE THERE ISN'T A SECURITY CAMERA PRESENT (UNLESS, OF COURSE, YOU DON'T MIND!).

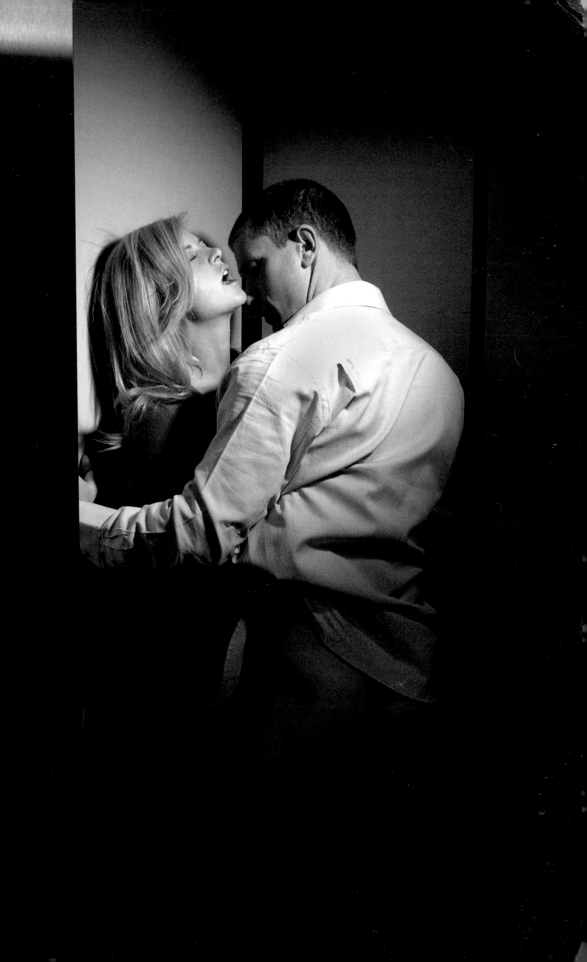

"He reached under my skirt and pulled down my panties while setting my legs apart with his foot, like in a police arrest."

And sometimes it is a noontime romp that amps up the heat, as one woman in her mid-forties confessed:

"I was at the computer checking my messages when I heard the downstairs door close. At first I was startled because I wasn't expecting anyone. The next thing I heard was an almost thunderous pounding of someone coming up the stairs growling. I got really scared. I could feel my heart pounding against my chest. Then I saw him and my fear turned to lust. It was my husband, a cop, stopping by for a 'lunchtime snack.'

"I turned to face him and he gripped my shoulders to make me stand and face the wall, arms up and opened. He reached under my skirt and pulled down my panties while setting my legs apart with his foot, like in a police arrest. Then he started to frisk me and before I could catch my breath he had his hand between my legs moving back and forth around my clit. He was breathing in my neck and telling me how much he wanted me. I was so turned on I thought I would pass out."

Apparently, this cop's wife also knows how to make use of an opportunity. Here's how she used her husband's off-duty assignment to her advantage:

"My husband was upstairs at a high-priced tech store observing for shoplifters. The owner had complained that he was losing a lot of the smaller items in his store to kids and some adults. The police suggested a camera surveillance system. After all, it was a tech shop, but the owner insisted he wanted a live surveillance so that word would get around about an immediate arrest.

"I was hanging out with my husband for a few minutes, observing through a one-way glass. He was standing behind me and I reached back and started massaging his crotch. He could see the sly smile on my face reflected in the glass and immediately got rock hard. I immediately got wet. He lifted my dress and slipped himself into me from behind. He held me close to him with one hand and rubbed my clit with the other. All the while we were watching the people below and also watching ourselves in the reflection of the glass. When I came I screamed so loud that people downstairs were looking around the store."

The woman above is certainly not alone when it comes to mixing pleasure with work. Another woman, just turning thirty, added her experience:

"My fantastic quickie begins with online flirting. I love to type in graphic descriptions and get some really sexy notes from my boyfriend. We work in different departments at the same place and we live nearby. Every once in a while we get so worked up that we both duck out of work, go home and have sex that, while it only lasts for a few minutes, feels so good and makes me want more! And I think it has the fear thing attached because we have to go back to work afterward. I'm sure the others at work have their suspicions; we both have this gleam in our eyes that we simply can't hide."

Do You Have the Quickie Mindset?

I'm not making this stuff up. In a survey conducted by Bowling Green State University, a group of men and women, ages twenty-five to forty-three, were asked, "If you had one choice—and you could have only one—which would you choose: hard, driving, fast sex or slow, gentle sex?" The majority of the women chose hammer city.

Who are these women? They're women just like you, except for one thing, one very important thing. They have attitude, and not just any attitude, but a string of beliefs that ignites their sexuality. I've met them, and talked to quite a few over the years. Here's what I've learned about them.

TOP TEN ATTITUDES OF WOMEN WHO LOVE QUICKIES

1. **When it comes to sex drive, I'm behind the wheel.**
   Women who want to supercharge their sex engine don't wait around patiently for a jump. Instead, they fuel up with sex-boosting strategies that heighten their sensuality. They give themselves permission to conjure up fantasies and don't believe in mind police—they allow themselves to be bad girls in their mind's eye. "My fantasies are those of a secret slut that lives in my head, and I love her!" one woman told me.

2. **It's not about perfection for me.**
   A hot babe doesn't waste time in front of the mirror fretting about cellulite or wishing she looked like a starving model, skinny and child-like. Instead, she sees herself as a healthy, full-fledged woman loaded with sensual capabilities. "When I walk into a room full of men, I walk in like I own it," a woman in her mid-forties confessed. "And it's not because I'm gorgeous," she added. "I could probably lose a few pounds, but I'm not about to torture myself with that like so many women do."

3. **I know I've got it.**
   A woman who believes in herself and feels sexy turns on men. Some women get that, and others don't; those who don't are too inhibited to dress sexy, act sexy, or allow themselves to feel sexy. Guys may initially be attracted to Ms. Hot Body, but if she doesn't have that inner sex appeal his interest quickly wanes. As one woman said, "My guy knows I'm hot because I know I'm hot and I'm not afraid to flaunt it."

   Sex appeal doesn't burst on the scene automatically. You need to do something to feel something. So how do you start? Fake it until you make it. That's what Merri did. A twenty-eight-year-old editor, Merri dressed like a banker and didn't dare let her inner slut even come close to surfacing. She had a world-class crush on a literary agent she lunched with from time to time.

   Nothing was happening with her Girl Scout persona so she started imagining letting that inner slut make an appearance. After a glass of wine, she leaned toward him and let her eyes do the talking. Six months of incredible action later, she still hasn't reined in that attitude.

4. **I'm willing and able to ask for what I want in the sack.**
   It's ironic, some women are monsters in business and passive in bed. Your guy wants to please you; after all, his ego is on the line big-time. He's been socialized

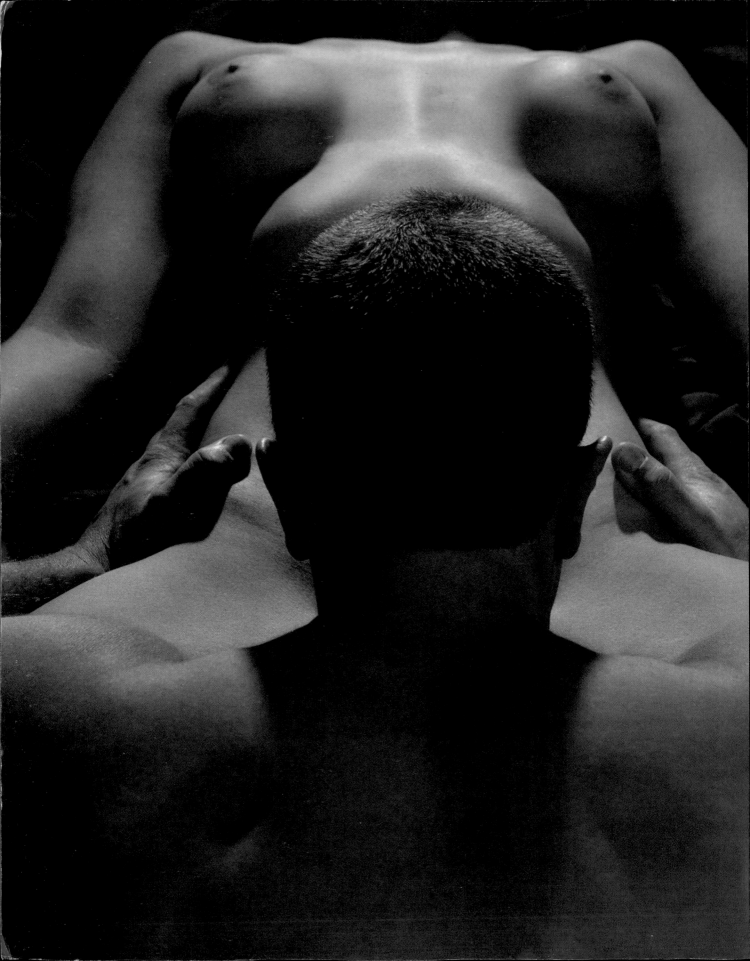

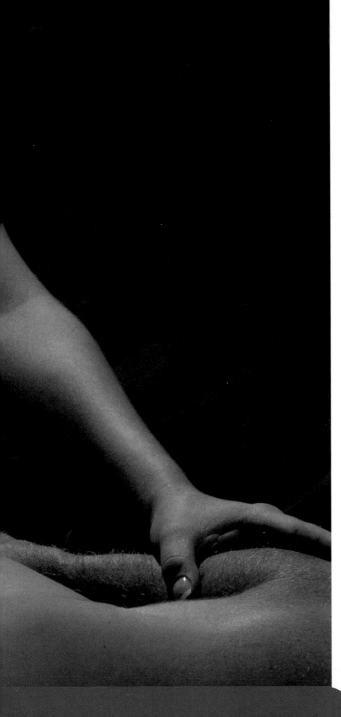

to strive to be the world's greatest lover. Yet he doesn't read minds, especially in the sack. Women who are into sex tell their partners how they like to be touched.

If you're not used to being so forward sexually, start by praising his sexual performance. Compliment him on what he does do well, then add a subtle (okay, not so subtle) suggestion, such as "I get crazy when you go down on me." One woman, in her late thirties, put it this way: "I'm simply not going to let my partner's expectations or the fear of looking silly stop me from asking for what I crave. That's teen stuff, I'm past that."

5. **My orgasm is as important to me as it is to you.**

Women who are into sex are like men; their orgasm counts. Come on, how many guys view their orgasm as optional? They view their orgasm as part of the deal, and women who are sexual beings share their attitude. It's not about entitlement, it's about expectation; kind of like success, if you anticipate it, it is more likely to occur. If you feel you don't deserve it, chances are you'll get just what you deserve—nothing.

Sexual satisfaction, like many things in life, is a self-fulfilling prophecy. If you don't expect to explode with ecstasy it won't happen. So start believing that every-time orgasms aren't elusive rewards reserved for a few select women—they're yours for the taking.

ORAL SEX FOR WOMEN
ORAL SEX FOR WOMEN, OR CUNNILINGUS, IS AN ART WITHIN ITSELF. IT IS A SIGNIFICANT PART OF BRINGING A WOMAN TO ORGASM, AND REQUIRES DELICATE SKILL, PATIENCE, PRACTICE, AND DEDICATION.

6. **I make it a point to get really good at one thing.**

Women who are sexual gurus are not good at everything. That's unrealistic. In any area of life no one is going to master everything. But getting good at one thing, so good that you can improvise and vary that one thing so that it looks like you're good at a lot of things, is the path to becoming an artist.

Being a master of one naughty move can morph you from a routine hot-and-heavy lover to world-class status. And you don't have to do something exceptional, your signature style can be about invoking an entire mood: spontaneous, daring, and dirty. "Guys may not be naturally sensual," a woman in her thirties told me, "but I can make 'sensual' so erotic it drives him wild."

7. **I know and follow the principle of reciprocity.**

Sexually charged women know that what goes around eventually comes around. They are attentive, sensuous, and sexually generous. It pays off. Guys who get what they want do their best to give back what you want. There's nothing hotter than a grateful guy. Having a willing woman to explore his secret desires blows him away and he's going to do his best to explore yours.

Taking the time to experiment with new caresses and positions doesn't just make your guy grovel, it pays you back in spades. "It's not that way with all guys," a twenty-something woman told me. "But I'm not interested in all guys," she continued, "just those that share my erotic generosity."

8. **I treat sex like a movie with great sequels.**

There are just so many times the same movie keeps your interest. But if the sequel really rocks, the story stays alive. Women who are sexual keep the story moving along; they're great sequel writers. As soon as sex loses its erotic edge, the "in-the-know babes" take fast action. They'll change locations, get ideas from steamy videos, bring in a third party in the form of a sex toy, or pull something close to the edge, such as acting out a secret fantasy or test-driving a scorching new position.

Hot babes keep the heat turned up high by bringing variety—and welcoming their guy's attempt to bring variety—to their sex play. A typical goal of a naughty babe is to bring something playful yet new to her pleasure nest as often as possible. The key is to keep the mischief in and the boredom out.

9. **I'm for sexual equality.**

Hot babes know that sexism puts people in simplistic and limiting categories. (The man should initiate sex. The woman should be submissive. Sex on the edge is a male thing, and so forth.) "Being bold about sex is not exclusive to men," a woman in her mid-thirties insisted. "Sex doesn't have to be the right time or the right place, and it doesn't have to be the guy's initiative," she said. Women who are very sexual don't think narrowly about sex.

10. I don't take sex all that seriously.

Women who love sex don't fuss; they take sex lightly. Sex is supposed to be fun, and sometimes it's funny too. "I was having this really raunchy romp with a younger guy one afternoon and I fell out of the bed," a woman approaching fifty said. "It was an awkward moment and for a second I looked up from the floor with a feeling of embarrassment, then I burst out laughing. He did too. We ended up having one hell of a memorable afternoon."

These women also don't get caught up in life's hassles. Rather than use hard times as excuses to pass on sex, they see them as opportunities to light up their lives with passion. They know that skin-to-skin contact is what they need for what ails them. It's about living and loving, not whining and withdrawing.

Putting off pleasure because of life's annoyances just doesn't wash for the sexual woman. The truly sexual woman knows that even if she's not wildly turned on, she's doing herself a favor by slipping into a sensuous state of mind.

"Being a master of one naughty move can morph you from a routine hot-and-heavy lover to world-class status."

FIVE REASONS TO DO IT NOW!

1. **PERK UP!** Grabbing a quickie is a superior mood lifter to Prozac; it works faster, feels way better, and there's no chance of weight gain.

2. **STAY HOT!** There's no better way to jump-start your inner slut (without drugs!) than by keeping your body primed for action. According to research by Eileen Palace, Ph.D., director of the Center for Sexual Health in New Orleans, by increasing the stimulation your body receives, you are priming yourself to be more easily receptive to additional stimulation. It's the opposite of "use it or lose it." Fast and dirty leads to being more receptive to the same. Sex begets more sex. Studies show that lovemaking elevates the levels of brain chemicals associated with desire. So the best way to increase your yearning for sex is to have it.

3. **SLEEP DEEP!** Quickies get the job done, and you still get a decent night's sleep. What's more, there's nothing bad about falling asleep smiling. It's all good!

4. **CREATE GOODWILL!** Novelty, the forbidden, and being aroused by the unknown are important contributors that lead men to stray. Why stray when he has that with you? Surprising him with sex on the run will help keep him faithful. Besides, you're creating goodwill you can collect on when you need that special favor.

5. **RAISE THE FLAME!** Okay, quickies are not the new miracle cure to save a relationship that's already taken a major nosedive. But if you're used to sex in the same way (him on top?), at the same time (Saturday night?), and in the same place (bed?), breaking that pattern with a quickie when you're stuck in that traffic jam is definitely going to notch up the passion. That is precisely the role of the quickie— boredom prevention with extras. What's more, the glow lasts. One poll found that couples who speed up sex will kiss, touch, and cuddle more.

That is precisely the role of the quickie—boredom prevention with extras.

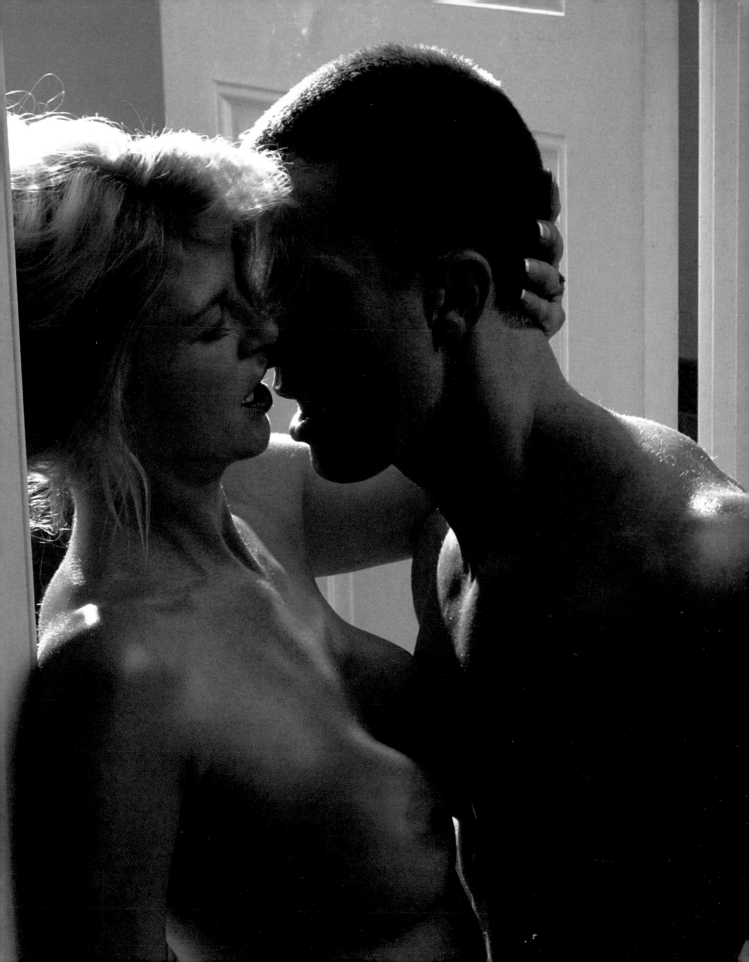

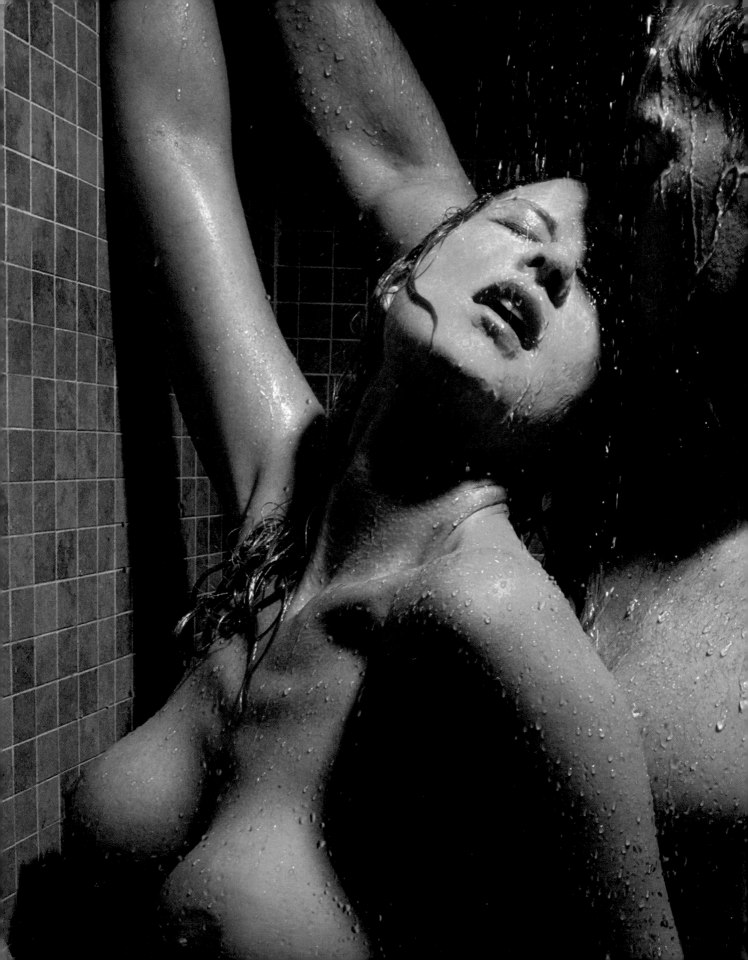

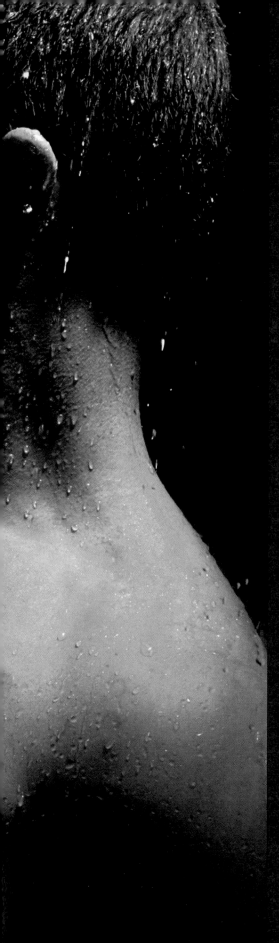

2

Quickie Warm-Ups

The Building Blocks of Passion

There is a time and place for almost everything we do in life, and often there is the long version and the short version. You normally sleep a full night, but you also might take short naps. You usually sit down to a full meal, but when pressed you might skip the meal and stop at the corner for a double shot espresso on the run. An argument might be made in favor of eating a full meal instead of skimping and loading up on caffeine. After all, how nourishing is a container of coffee? And that's the argument against quickies: not enough nourishment.

My view is that once in a while it's not a bad idea to skip the nourishment and go for the energy blast. Breaking the routine on occasion is a good thing. But making quickies a routine thing is not the way to go.Creating the right mood for lovemaking is often stated to be the path to heightened pleasure, and generally this is true. But the couple who waits for the mood to be right every time may miss out on all but their self-imposed notions of "romantic" sex. It's too limiting.

Quickie sex often has a quality all its own. Within the confines of your loving relationship it is neither more nor less worthwhile or trivial than lovemaking that has been carefully considered and conforms to the conventional.

Here are some beginning quickie scenarios. Remember, they may not always be quick (although any of my suggestions can be abbreviated), but they're different. Each one brings a touch of variety and a bit of the less conventional. Like spices in cooking, some people respond to a hint and others need a large dollop before they experience a new sensation. We're beginning with a hint; in the "recipes" to come we'll ramp up the spice.

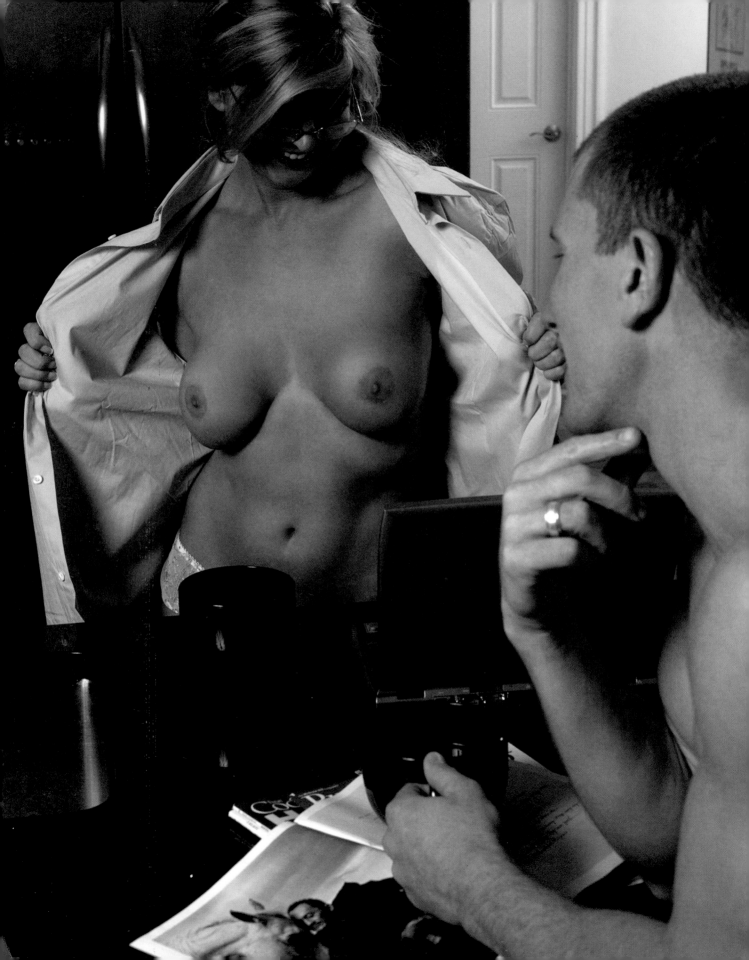

STRETCHING YOUR SEXUAL BOUNDARIES

1. **EACH MORNING,** before the two of you get up, spend just a couple of minutes getting each other stimulated. Orgasm is not the point; it's about the tease, creating something to take with you in your mind's eye through the day.

2. **HAVE SEX** somewhere you might not usually have it, but in your own home. Try some of the following locations:
Shower. Great for oral sex. The water gently trickling over the head and shoulders of the partner kneeling at the other's genitals adds to the pleasure.
Living room. You can have sex sitting in a chair, on the sofa, the floor, maybe the coffee table. A fireplace in winter adds ambiance, and candlelight works, too.
Kitchen. Floor, table, counters. If your guy is tall, you can have intercourse sitting on the counter while he stands.
Dining room. Chairs, table, floor. The association with food can make sex more interesting, especially if the table hasn't been cleared.
Garage. Have you ever made love on the hood of a parked car? Make sure the hood isn't hot and you don't have one of those motion sensitive alarms! Look around the garage for other ideas. Improvise.

3. **ARRIVE SOMEWHERE TEN MINUTES EARLY.** Stay in the car and stimulate each other for ten minutes only. Don't be late.

4. **SURPRISE EACH OTHER** with a few minutes of oral sex. Alternate turns.

5. **TEASE EACH OTHER.** You're dressed, running ten minutes late, hurrying out the door. Your partner is still getting dressed or lingering over his breakfast. On your way out, flash him. Yes, *flash him.* Quickly expose your breast and hike up your skirt to show some leg.

6. **DON'T TAKE OFF YOUR CLOTHES.** Remember when you and your guy first got involved? That primal, animalistic groping? Remember being so desperate for your lover's body that you didn't take the time to remove clothing, only pushed aside the necessary items? Start kissing on the sofa (or in the car) and recapture those feelings.

7. **COMBINE FOOD AND SEX.** Even adults like to occasionally play with their food. Take food to bed with you and feed each other. Get more creative. For example, melt some chocolate, apply it liberally to each other's body, and lick it off. Chocolate is not only delicious, it contains phenyl ethylamine, a mood-boosting chemical that can incite lust.

8. **PAINT YOUR BODIES.** Use water soluble finger paints or body paints—some come flavored—to decorate one another's nude bodies. Paint yourself to look like the members of primitive tribes and make love the way you imagine they do.

BREAST FLASH

SEX SHOULD BE PLAYFUL AND FUN. TEASING KEEPS IT LIGHT AND FRESH.

CHOCOLATE FOREPLAY

INCORPORATING FOOD INTO FOREPLAY CAN BE EXTREMELY EROTIC. SHARING A "MIDNIGHT SNACK" COULD PROVE MORE SATISFYING THAN YOU EXPECTED.

foreplay

EXPLORING: PHONE SEX, BONDAGE, AND LIGHT S/M

Almost anything that takes a couple out of the same-time, same-place, same-way routine adds excitement to lovemaking. A move as simple as turning on the lights can create change. Here are some less conventional, alternative forms of love play.

Phone Sex

If you haven't looked at a sex magazine in recent years, you probably would be more surprised at the pages of phone-sex ads than at the nude layouts. Men have always been aroused by sex talk because it creates strong visual images in the mind. The phone sex industry was developed to fulfill an unmet need.

If either you or your partner travel on business—or even if you don't—phone sex is a way to generate enthusiasm for the coming reunion. Here's how to play the game.

1. **WARM UP** by leaving erotic messages on his voice mail—assuming no one else has access to the messages, of course. Don't feel guilty about talking dirty. "Nice" girls weren't raised to graphically talk about sex, and that's exactly what makes your comments so exciting when they come out of your mouth intended for his ears only. Your voice is an arousal too, just like mouths, lips, tongues, hands, and genitals.

2. **LEARN** some new words. Erotic novels are filled with a variation of words for genitals. The steamier romance novels are another good source of inspiration. You may also want to check out *Vox*, Nicholson Baker's novel about phone sex. (It's a quick read!)

3. **PRACTICE.** If the words don't come easy to you, say them out loud when you're alone. Get used to the feel of using graphic words. Like learning a foreign language, dirty talk takes some practice.

4. **RENT MOVIES** you consider erotic—and listen to them. Close your eyes so you won't be distracted by the visual content of the film. You'll be surprised at how much the words, tone of voice, and inflection contribute to the experience.

5. **READ EROTICA** out loud to each other. You may find it easier to be creative on your own after reading other scripts. Choose novels with a lot of dialogue.

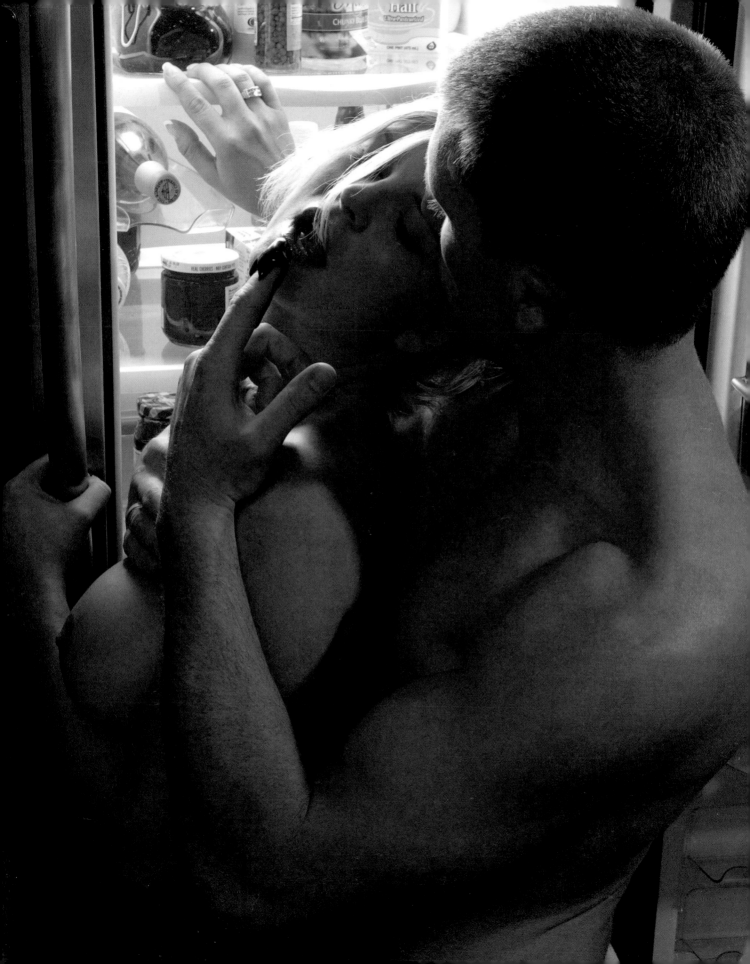

6. **NOW YOU'RE READY** for phone sex. Choose a scenario that you know will be particularly arousing to your partner. Phone-sex operators say that anal sex, oral sex, and female domination scenarios are the most popular with their callers. Remember to be specific. The heat of phone sex is in the details.

7. **ADD SOUND EFFECTS.** Heavy breathing, panting, and soft moans add a note of similitude to the experience.

8. **WHEN YOU'RE MORE COMFORTABLE** with the game, create scenarios out of your own unexpressed desires and hidden fantasies. Phone sex with your lover is a safe way to explore your inner slut.

9. **WHEN YOU'RE REALLY COMFORT-ABLE,** you may want to masturbate during phone sex—or maybe not, you may want to leave the mental excitation at a peak and wait to see him in person.

Bondage

Bondage is erotic restraint, the sensual experience of safe captivity. Light bondage, or "tie and tease," may be the most common sex game couples play. One partner ties the other, either lightly binding wrists together or binding wrists and sometimes ankles to the bedposts. The bound partner is then "helpless" and must submit to the other's sexual desires. The object of the game is intensifying pleasure through delaying gratification. The one in charge teases the other to the brink of orgasm, pulls back, and teases again.

How to proceed:

> Using silk scarves or ties or Velcro restraints (purchased in a sex-toy catalogue or store), loosely bind your partner's wrists and/or ankles. If he is comfortable with it, add a blindfold.

> Check the bindings to make sure they are not constricting blood flow.

> Kiss, caress, stroke, and fondle his body, avoiding genitals.

> Using oral and manual stimulation, stimulate him to a level of high arousal.

> Abruptly stop genital stimulation.

> Again, kiss, caress, stroke, and fondle, avoiding the genitals.

> Repeat the stop-start method of genital stimulation until your partner begs for an orgasm.

> Remember, even light bondage can lead to muscle cramps. You don't want to sustain the experience so long that your partner is begging for a massage, not an orgasm!

QUICKIE

LIGHT BONDAGE

LIGHT BONDAGE CAN BE USED AS AN OCCASIONAL FORM OF EROTIC PLAY TO BREAK UP YOUR SEXUAL ROUTINE AND SPICE THINGS UP.

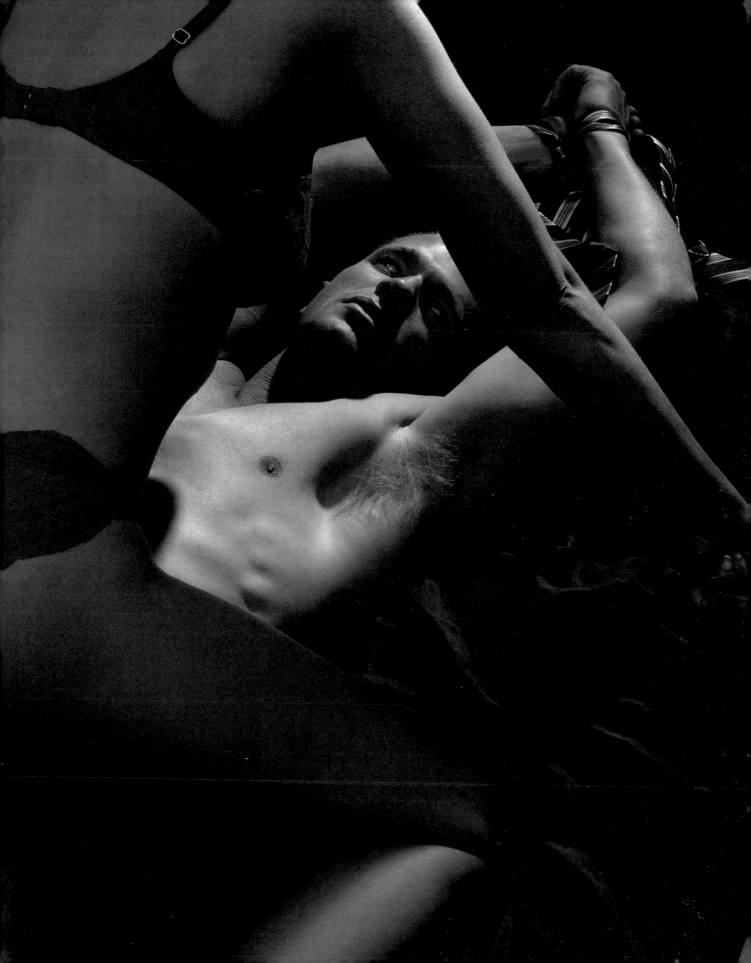

Light S/M

More theater than pain, light S/M (sadomasochism) games are erotic power exchanges between consenting partners. They sometimes involve costumes and props and nearly always include role-playing. One partner plays the dominant, the other the submissive character in an erotic drama. The dominant controls the action by administering light doses of physical pain and/or verbal abuse and making the submissive do some sexual bidding. The submissive is really in charge, however, because it is understood between players that the game doesn't go any further than the submissive desires. The word sadomasochism is derived from combining "sadist," one who enjoys inflicting pain and/or humiliation on others, and "masochist," one who enjoys receiving pain and/or humiliation. People who take this behavior to extremes are a small minority. For them, the exchange of pain has almost or entirely replaced sexual activity. They refer to S/M as a lifestyle because it does define how they live their lives. The vast majority of people who dabble in S/M, however, use it as an occasional form of erotic play to break their routine and intensify arousal and orgasm. They are "switch players," alternating the dominant and submissive roles.

If you want to play, here are the guidelines:

> Don't underestimate the importance of costumes and props. Certain themes of clothing, type of fabric or other materials, and special accoutrements have S/M connotations. Visit a sex-toy shop or browse a catalogue for ideas. Generally these props include tight-fitting leather or rubber garments, anything of the color black, bustiers, corsets, garter belts, stockings, very high heels or pumps, boots, masks, nipple clamps, bondage gear, and spanking implements.

> Work from a script. You don't have to write down the dialogue, but it helps to have a plot worked out before beginning. Talk in detail with your partner about what you want to do.

> Set limits and stick to them. A velvet-covered whip can sting. So can words. Be clear about how far is too far to go, both verbally and physically.

> Use a safe word. The submissive should be able to stop the game at any time by saying the safe word. Don't use "no." It's too confusing.

> Remember that a little goes a long way. You may fantasize giving or receiving a level of rough treatment that would be a turnoff in real life.

> Be sure your partner is aroused before you administer pain, and be sure your partner continues to be aroused by the action.

> Switch roles the next time you play.

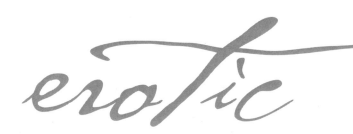

SIX TIPS FOR GETTING STARTED

Breaking the routine, as we've seen, can be as simple as turning on the lights or groping in the car, or it could involve something more elaborate, such as a loosely scripted S/M or bondage game. In any case, to keep up the heat, use the following suggestions:

1. **DRESS FOR THE OCCASION.** Slip into something lacy. According to one survey, guys who fail to notice that you're wearing glasses or that you shaved your head (well, not quite), literally leap to attention at the sight of some lacey underwear.

2. **PEEK AT A SNAP.** Keep a naked picture of your guy, or maybe of the two of you in a very compromised position, in your wallet. Peek at it during a business meeting, while you're on the phone, or whenever else it's not quite the right time. You'll feel flirty and dirty all day.

3. **INTRODUCE A THIRD PARTY.** There's nothing like your own personal buzz-in-a-rush joystick to speed things up. Not sure which one to get? Check out the Resources section for my recommendation of the best of the best. Using a battery operated model when you're not near an electrical outlet will ensure that you don't run out of juice before yours starts to flow.

4. **HAVE SEX IN PUBLIC WITHOUT RISK.** A woman I spoke with told me about something she tried that's really cool: Before going out for the evening she handed a small black plastic box, about the size of a pack of gum, to her guy. He put the box in his pocket, and off they went.

    The little box contains batteries and has a button her guy presses whenever the mood strikes. Maybe he holds it down a few moments and shoots a mischievous glance at her. It's naughty.

Here's how it works: Imagine a pair of thong panties. The sort of elastic, G-string thingie you might expect some hot number to wear on a beach in the French Riviera. Only in the place on the thong where there would typically be a tiny triangle of fabric, there is a flat piece of soft purple plastic molded in the shape of a butterfly. It's about a half-inch thick with perhaps a four-inch wingspan at its widest point, and there is a plastic tail at the bottom that curves backward and upward, protruding about one inch.

Inside this plastic butterfly is a tiny electric motor and a receiver. Depressing the button on the small black plastic box, which is a wireless remote control with a range of twenty-five feet, activates the receiver. Upon such activation, the motor causes the butterfly to vibrate.

It's not so quiet that it would be inaudible in a board meeting, but it's more than quiet enough to be employed covertly in a bar, in a movie theater, or at a party.

5. **CARRY A QUICKIE KIT.** Keep condoms and any props (silk scarves, handcuffs, etc.), lubrication, and your favorite sex toys on hand so that your naughty moments aren't stalled due to technicalities. Besides, just knowing that the equipment is in your presence may prompt dirty thoughts.

6. **WINK, WINK.** You're sitting in a restaurant, you give him a look that he recognizes and then you get up and walk toward the restroom. He gets up and follows you knowing full well what you're up to—he recognizes that look because the two of you have created your own quickie signal. It conveys, in no uncertain terms, **"You, me, here, now."**

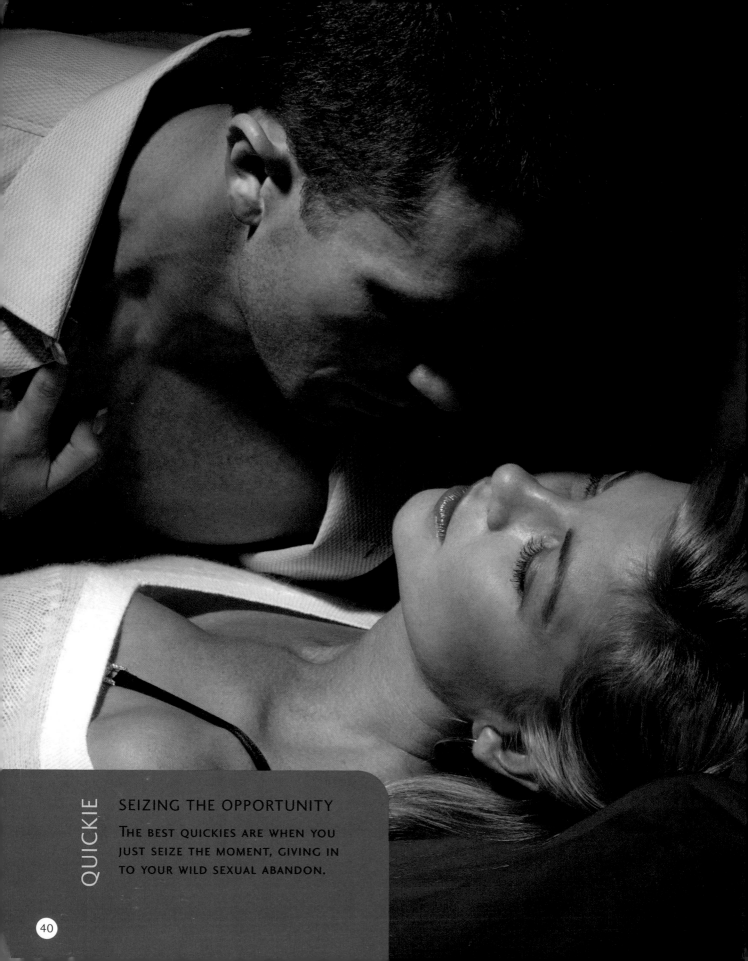

QUICKIE

SEIZING THE OPPORTUNITY

The best quickies are when you just seize the moment, giving in to your wild sexual abandon.

QUICKIE
WEEKEND GETAWAY

Your folks take the kids, and you take off—just the two of you for two days in a cabin, far from everyone and everything.

You stop off for dinner at an Italian restaurant right off the road. While he orders, you excuse yourself. In the ladies' room, you remove your underpants and put them in your purse.

The waiter takes your order as a pianist begins to play and a few diners take their places on the tiny dance floor. You slide your foot out of your shoe and let it rub against your partner's leg. He is startled at first, and then reaches under the table for your knee. You slide down a little in your seat and sigh, letting him know how much you enjoy this. His hand moves along the curve of your thigh, finally reaching its destination. He gasps as he feels the warm, heavy wetness between your legs.

When he has raised you to such a fever pitch that you're ready to scream, you push back your chair and pull him onto the dance floor. The two of you melt together—every pore, every cell is attached to him in some way. He holds you so close you can feel his erection pressing against your leg. "I want to make you come," he whispers.

You ask for the dinners to be wrapped; something has come up and you have to go. He guns the engine and you arrive at the cabin laughing hysterically, piling out of the car and running inside. You are about to tear off your clothes when he asks, almost guiltily, "Will you strip for me?"

You click on the radio by the bed, tuning the dial until you find an oldies station. The wail of an alto sax is all the incentive you need. You gyrate slowly, turning so that he can see all of you. You whirl around, and your silk skirt lifts with your motion, giving a glimpse of flesh before you let it drop. You undo the tie at his neck, and then loosen your sheer blouse to give a hint of cleavage.

He is getting clearly impatient and reaches into his travel bag. You can hear a faint mechanical humming as he comes toward you, holding something behind his back.

"What are you doing?" you ask, but then he slides the vibrator under your skirt, and you feel as though you're going to faint. You clutch him, and he runs the device along the front of your body to circle your nipples. It is alive and it makes them stand at attention, straining against the light silk. You take the toy from him, easing it down the front of his pants. He holds you close so that you can both benefit from its pulsing rhythm.

Still partly clothed, you come together, unable to wait any longer. The moon is high now, and the call of an owl reminds you how late it is. But this is your time together, and nothing is going to get in the way. You rip at each other's remaining clothes and he pulls you out to the little dock that connects the cabin with the lake. Are there others out there that might see you? It occurs to you but you just smile mischievously.

Entangled and surrounded by the warm, lapping water he licks your breasts and works his way down between your legs. His mouth is a hungry beast. "Too good," you groan and arch your hips, pressing forward, gaining the contact you crave, but his tongue dances, caressing you, taunting you, until you can't handle it any longer and explode. And when you say "more," he obeys you without a thought.

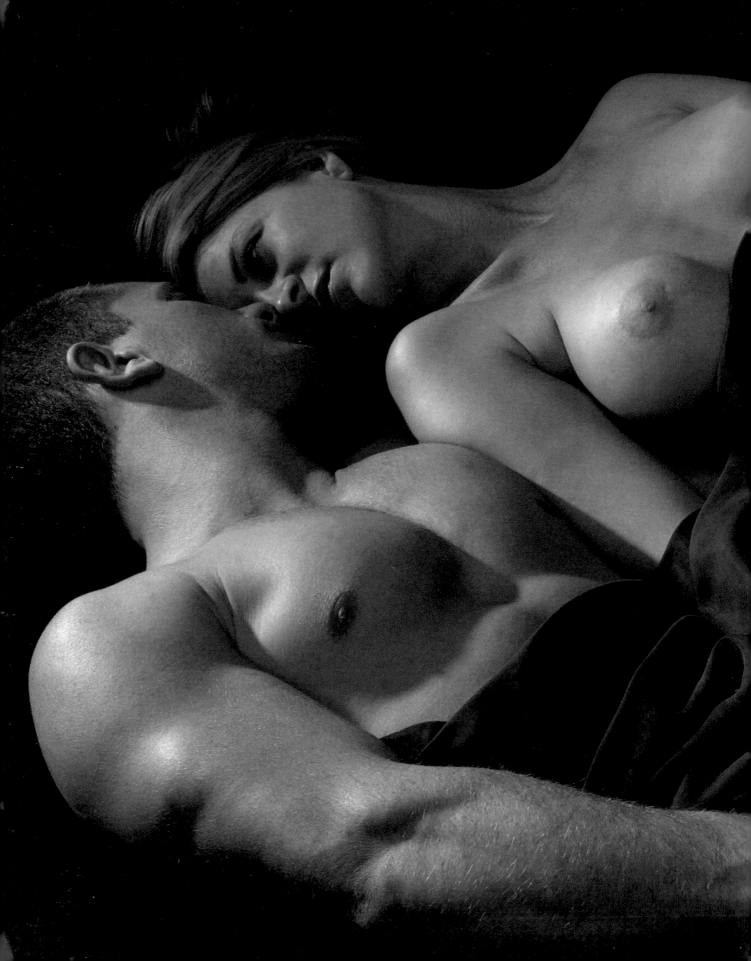

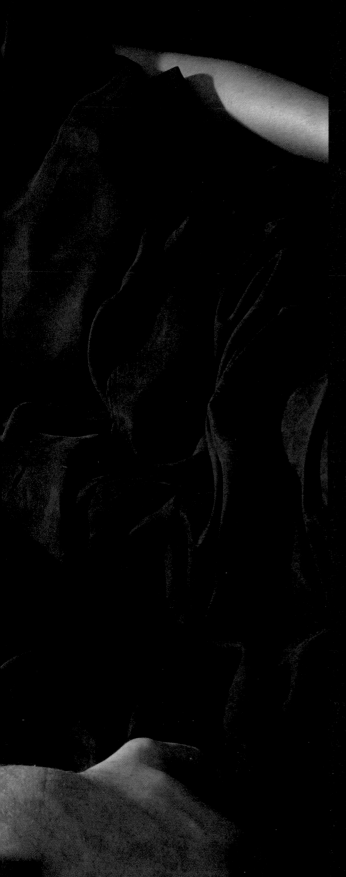

3

Peeking Over the Edge

THE SET-UP

So when is it appropriate to engage in quickie sex? Absolutely any chance you get—as long as you're using reasonable (albeit daring) judgment. The whole point of quickie sex is taking advantage of, or creating opportunity.

Why not wake up in the morning to something that's more refreshing than freshly squeezed orange juice? Indulge in a quick morning sex-fix and you'll notice a little spring in your step throughout the remainder of the day. The dishes can wait. Be late for work. Just don't be late every day, unless the guy rubbing up against you in the morning is the guy who signs your check. There's always later in the day, at home. But having sex in your own place, NOT in the bed, is only an appetizer, meant to whet your desire. As we've seen, there are unconventional games to play, phone sex, bondage, light S/M, and the like.

Still want more? You're a candidate for the advanced course: the fast and fabulous pleasures of the forbidden and the unexpected. Welcome to the world of outdoor orgasms, quickie hot spots, innovative foreplay, and the less traveled paths to carnal bliss.

First, dress for the part. Your guy has this view of you as being all about romance. And you do love romance, there's nothing wrong with that. But just because you are fundamentally hungry for romance doesn't mean you don't also want to be naughty.

How can he tell when you are in the mood to reenact a Mickey Rourke movie? He'll pay attention to what you're wearing. If you're sporting a low-cut top with a push-up bra and heels, a skirt that flows when you walk, the kind that's easy to get under, he'll get the hint that you've probably had wild sex in the back of your mind since you opened your eyes that morning (especially if you gave him that look of lust when you turned to him).

Just ask Paula, thirty-one. "When I'm in the mood for something wild, when I'm in bold mode, I definitely dress the part," she said. "I'm suggestive, big-time. I flirt with my eyes and I flaunt it. No way is it not going to register with him. He'd have to be blind and dumb, not my kind of guy."

Obviously, you want to encourage his full collaboration in your bad behavior with every bone in your body. So begin the tease and continue with every opportunity. Sneak your hand playfully between his knees under the table, unbutton his shirt button in the cab and swipe your hand sensually across his chest, or grab him from behind as he walks up the stairs.

When you're alone, do something you've never done before—whether it's tying a blindfold around his eyes or slipping a hand down the front of his pants, but not all the way—simply send the message that wild is just around the corner and closing in. Your inner slut is getting restless, but it's not quite time.

For now, it's about the tease, building up the tension. Each move is quick and dirty, nothing you do requires more time; it's about how you use the time you have. It's simply about being naughty and doing the unexpected until it makes him (and you!) feel like an out-of-control, lust-ridden animal.

LOCATION, LOCATION

Ask a real estate agent for her best advice about properties and you'll likely hear that it's all about one factor: location. The same can be true for sex. There's the bed at home, sure. There also are more creative locations at home, and then there's stepping up and out.

Stepping out where? That's up to you and your partner. It depends on your imagination and on your risk tolerance. My advice: Take a peek over the edge, but don't lean too far over unless you have bail money and are immune to embarrassment.

Here's a sampling of places to go, from the sublime to the frightening, and some reactions from women who've been there.

The Movies

Like other forms of entertainment, sometimes the action grabs you and sometimes you have to grab him to create your own action! That's what this twenty-nine-year-old woman did one rainy afternoon.

"When I was a teenager I worked in a movie theater for a few months. After having seen the same movie a few times I would get bored and my mind wandered. I often wandered to sexual thoughts, especially if the movie had some parts that were erotic. Then, one night I was watching a movie that was incredibly boring with my boyfriend of three years. One of the things I learned when I worked at the movies is that people rarely look backwards—and I took advantage of that. I sank down between the seats and gave him the most amazing oral sex. Then, he slipped down and did me. We watched a little more of the movie and then he rose up, put his coat over us and slipped into me while I did my best to pretend I was watching the screen. I would say that experience made the list of the best sex I ever had! I'll remember it forever and smile. The movie? Somehow I can't recall."

The Shower

Shower quickies are very common because of the privacy factor and, besides, it saves on hot water! Shower quickies work best when the element of surprise is added.

Here's what one woman, thirty-eight years old and divorced, said after her experience. "Recently while drying off from a bubble bath, my boyfriend came in with a very sly look on his face. He proceeded to take the towel from me and started kissing my neck. His kisses moved down my neck to my nipples while his hand moved between my legs. I was wet by now! He began massaging my clit while he kissed me on the lips and nipples and I had a major orgasm. Now I play with the idea of him sneaking up on me again and it gets me very hot!"

The Backyard

Yes, this is in and about your usual surroundings, but the usual can still be provocative—especially if privacy is not guaranteed. Listen to what Lisa, forty-one, experienced.

"We were out on the deck in the moonlight this past summer. We both had a couple of glasses of wine and I was feeling horny. My husband must have read my mind because he started taking his clothes off. I told him the neighbors were going to see him but he just smiled and continued. Seeing him there naked out in the open was beginning to make me wet. He got me to remove my shirt and bra first. He took it further and tried to get me out of my panties and shorts but I kept refusing. I was sitting on him facing away from him and could feel his erection, which was making me hornier. I was of two minds, one I was embarrassed about the possibility of someone seeing us, and the other I was excited about someone seeing us!

"Finally, I gave in to taking my shorts off. I was wearing a pair of thong panties so I could feel his penis against my lips. I was facing him on the chair and I had never made love that way. He

One of the things I learned when I worked at the movies is that people rarely look backwards—and I took advantage of that. I sank down between the seats and gave him the most amazing oral sex.

was trying his best to slip himself into me and I was very tempted, but I kept motioning to the door and whispering, 'Let's go inside.' He was persistent and I was getting more and more turned on. This makes me laugh, but he said he would just put it in a little—so typical. But I went along. I pulled my thong to the side and he slid right in. He felt incredible inside me in that position. At that point all thoughts about going back inside the house vanished. I was thrusting so hard I almost fell onto the deck. I had the most intense orgasm I had ever had. The next day my neighbor called me and thanked me for giving her and her husband the motivation to have the best sex they ever had. Yikes!"

The Beach

Sure, a hand job (mutual) is easy under a beach blanket, it seems movie-made for getting swept away. But when sand gets in those creases of the vulva it can cause irritations, so consider jumping in the water.

Making your own waves in the water can be super exciting because, well, just because. But the water needs to be reasonably warm so that his erection doesn't sink.

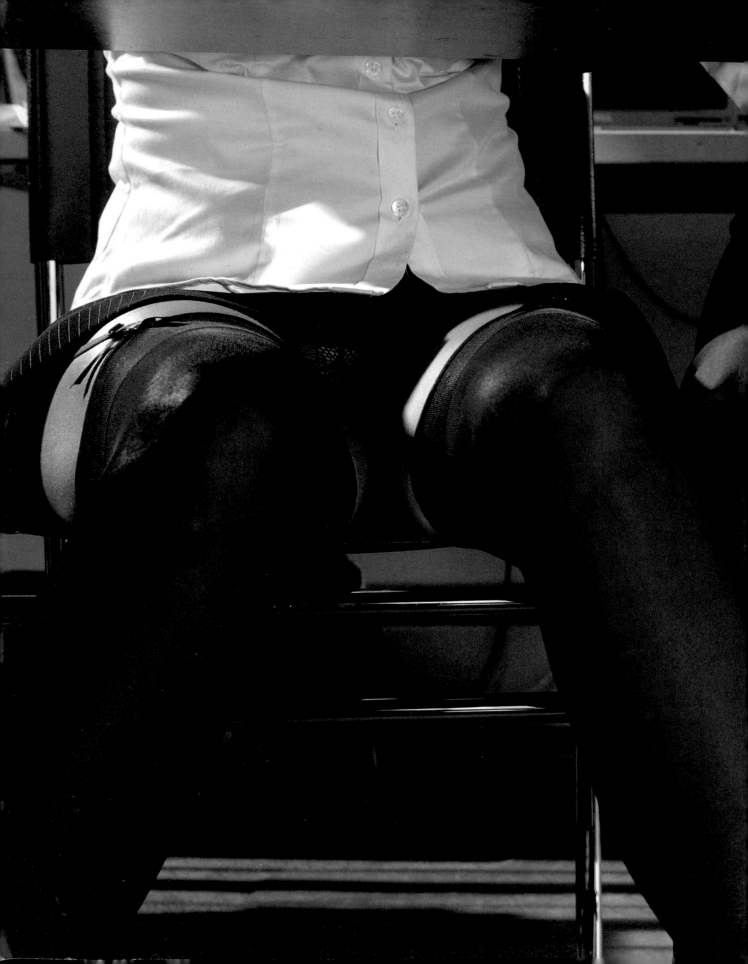

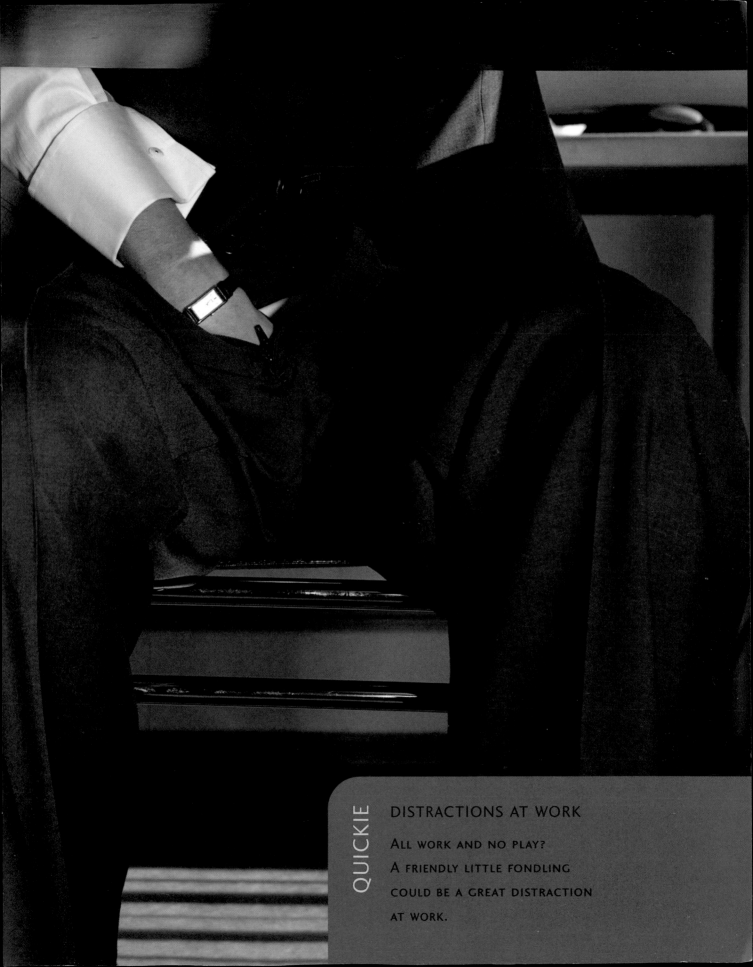

QUICKIE

DISTRACTIONS AT WORK

ALL WORK AND NO PLAY?
A FRIENDLY LITTLE FONDLING
COULD BE A GREAT DISTRACTION
AT WORK.

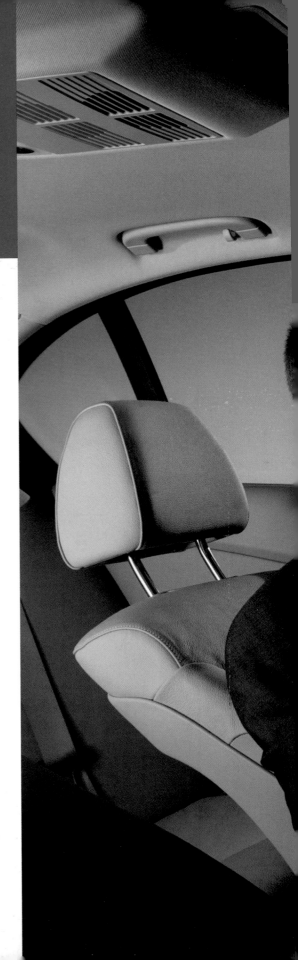

QUICKIE

CAR SEX

HAVING A QUICKIE IN YOUR CAR CAN BE A SEXUALLY EXPLOSIVE (AND LIBERATING) EXPERIENCE. IT'S PROBABLY BEST NOT TO ENGAGE IN THIS BLIND LUST WHILE YOU'RE DRIVING THOUGH.

One H_2O expert, a woman in her early forties who knows the secret of warm water, told me about her experiences.

"We've done this a few times on the beach with plenty of folk around. What we do is go into the water together and wade out until the water is well above waist level. Then my husband reaches down and slips his penis out of his swimming trunks. Shortly, I slip off my bikini bottom and give it to him to tuck into his trunks, trying to do all this inconspicuously! Then I wrap my legs around his torso, he slips inside me and we go at it. To anyone watching it would probably look like we're just kissing and making out. It's the kind of sex that just keeps giving; we think about and get turned on by it constantly."

The Car

Remember, if you indulge on the car, make sure the alarm is off and the engine is cool. Inside the car it is good practice to avoid an unintentional pressing of the horn—unless you are interested in having your picture taken with someone's cell phone!

While there's a lot to be said for driving a Porsche, it's not a frolic friendly vehicle. Hopefully, your car is larger. Of course, if you have a station wagon, SUV, or van, you're all set.

A woman who wouldn't give me her age (she looked great, but I'm not going to venture a guess in case she's reading this) told me a sexy story featuring her in the leading role.

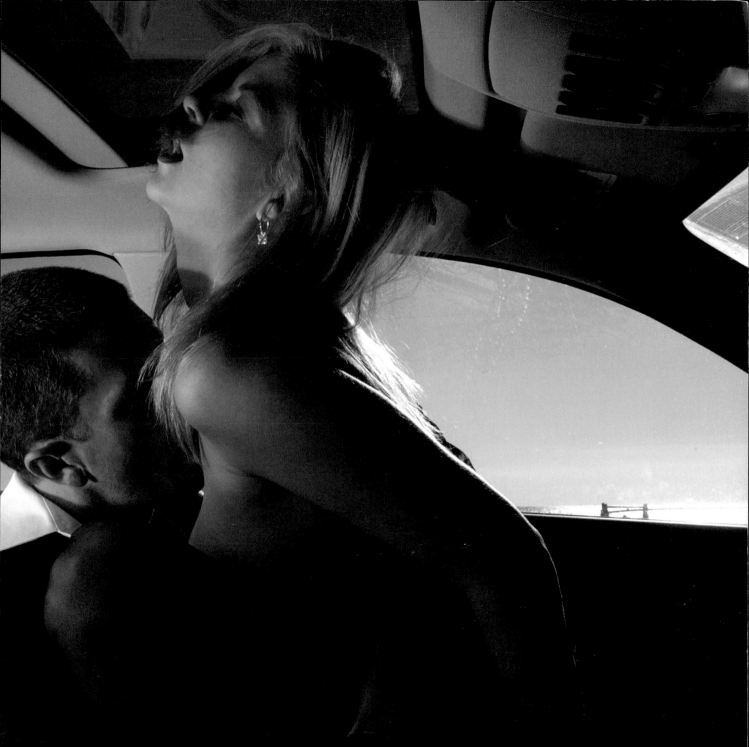

> *"The biggest risk yet was when he convinced me to sit on top of him and have sex right there on the side of a busy road."*

"We went to visit our friends upstate. On the way back home we made a two-hour drive into a four-hour adventure. It started out with my husband asking me to take off my shorts and drive bottomless. I glanced over at him and he had this really mischievous smirk on his face. 'I dare you,' he said. He didn't think that I would do it considering that I am a very shy person. I was in a frisky mood and pretty bored so I stepped out of character and told him I would take off my shorts if he did too. We fondled each other while I drove. It was very naughty, and very hot.

"We finally had to pull into a parking lot and get each other off. By the time we got back on the road it was dark and we took off our shorts again and started feeling each other. Once on the highway I took off my shirt and bra so I was driving with only my shoes on.

"My husband got so turned on he leaned over to kiss my breast while rubbing between my legs. I got distracted and immediately pulled off the road and had several orgasms. When we got on the road again we switched seats. As soon as he got back on the highway I started to go down on him, then I got so hot I wanted him inside me. No way were we going to do that while he was driving. As it was, we had already taken a chance. Not only did we compromise our own driving, I noticed that several drivers passing us were distracted as well, especially a truck driver who almost

drove off the road. The biggest risk yet was when he convinced me to sit on top of him and have sex right there on the side of a busy road. I'm not a very adventurous person, but THAT was very satisfying and exciting!"

The Office

It sounds like a bold maneuver but if guts are your glory and you don't depend on the job, or if you are looking for an unusual recommendation for another, then the office is for you! Here's one story that's reasonably tame, because the office where this thirty-something woman had her encounter belonged to her husband.

"We were having a screened porch added on to our house by my husband's work crew (he's a contractor). So I have all these hunky guys working bare-chested around the house. Even though they work for my husband—or maybe because they work for him—they didn't hesitate to flirt. One guy had these deep green eyes; I found myself panting after he looked at me! And all this is occurring while the sex between my husband and I over the past months was getting boring! That's it, I said to myself. I stopped by my husband's office with the excuse that I wanted to get some mail over to him. His office is very busy; it's a madhouse of activity with people running around all over the place. As soon as I came in I winked at him. This was no ordinary wink, this wink had power. Like, Wow! Now!

"He got it, or maybe he was having his own sexy thoughts because next thing I know we are on the floor of his office bathroom. My dress is up, and my panties are down at my ankles. His pants are down past his knees, and he's pumping his hard manhood deep inside me. He did me so hard I screamed out loud. Then in the background, we heard someone moving around in his office. It was his secretary and his son from his first marriage who is in partnership with him.

He left me on the floor of the bathroom and went outside to talk to his son. His son left before I came out. I will never know if his son knew I was in there getting 'serviced,' but his secretary gave me an awkward smile when I left. I kissed him on the cheek, gave him his mail and went home. That night, my husband went down on me, and I reciprocated. What a day!"

The Great Outdoors

Sunlight is prescription-free Viagra. One theory is that sunlight makes people hornier because it suppresses their melatonin, a hormone believed to be the biological equivalent of a full meal—in other words, sunlight leaves you feeling hungry and if you're in the right company the hunger isn't for food. Being out in the sun may even be a double threat: It's also speculated that sunshine increases serotonin and other hormones that take us into back-to-nature nookie.

Here's the experience of a thirty-five-year-old woman who may or may not understand the underlying biology of going at in the green, but she's definitely for it.

"My husband and I were hiking in the mountains. We went to an area pretty high up and clear where you could see for miles in every direction. He came up behind me and removed my backpack. He then ran his hands up my shirt and touched me with a very arousing intensity as he unhooked my bra. The feeling of him removing my bra and touching my nipples immediately got me very worked up. He took off my shirt and put it on a big boulder, turned me around, pulled down my hiking shorts, bent me over the boulder, and nailed me from behind. I'm not the type of woman who likes it that way, but that was Wow! Good thing no one else came up the trail because when I came it was with complete abandon. If someone were there, I don't think I could have stopped."

Other Places to Explore

There is nothing like a quickie in a friend's bathroom or public restroom to energize a relationship plagued by routine sex. Whether in a club or a restaurant, many couples have engaged in quickie sex in public bathrooms.

Also consider the clothing store changing room. It's not terribly surprising that some couples get hot watching one another change into different outfits—especially if the change is taking place somewhere other than in the privacy of their own home.

There's also the train, boat, plane, and if you live life in the fast lane, there's also the roller coaster and any other location your imagination and lust brings you to.

"*He took off my shirt and put it on a big boulder, turned me around, pulled down my hiking shorts, bent me over the boulder, and nailed me from behind.*"

orgasm

GETTING HOT AND BOTHERED IN RECORD TIME

1. **BE BOLD.** Place his hands where you want them, *on you*!

2. **WELCOME TENSION.** You often can be too relaxed in languorous sexual encounters. Orgasm is basically a tension release. Spontaneous quickies create tension that is sexually charged (unlike, for example, the tension of a tax audit!); consequently, the release is likely to be explosive.

3. **JUST DO IT!** Don't get caught in the details of the quickie. Couples who are into the once-in-a-while quickie have more sex because they have learned that each encounter doesn't need to have profound meaning. Sometimes it's just about a no-frills scratch for that itch.

4. **BRING HIM TO HIS KNEES.** Studies show a couple of minutes of oral sex (for you!) is a double feature: It will get you lubed and stimulated in all the right places at just the right pace.

5. **VERBALLY TEASE.** Make promises you aren't going to keep—yet. Tell him what you're going to do with his penis. Then make him wait until next time.

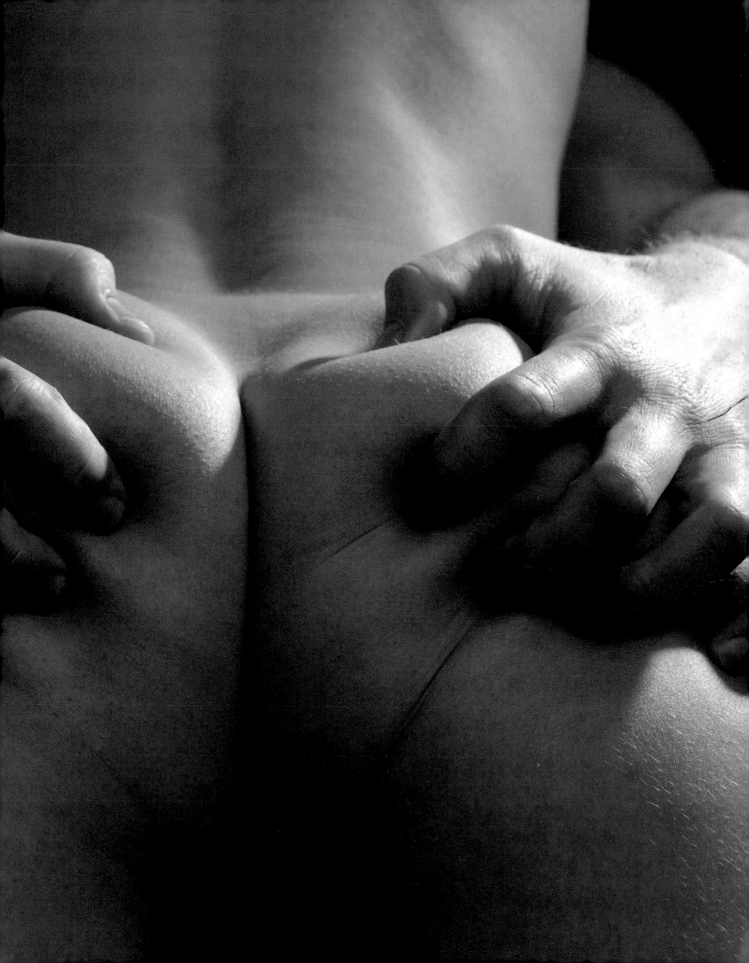

QUICKIE
AN UNFORGETTABLE SEND-OFF

He wanted everything to be perfect the night before you left for Belgium. He had started missing you the minute you told him you'd be doing research for three months. "I want to do something special for our last night— flowers, candles, soft music, whatever you'd like," he told you. But you just grinned. "I can think of something we'll both remember every day until I come back," you said. "My surprise."

You met outside your office and got in a cab just after rush hour had ended. It was chilly, and you clung together in the back seat. He was astounded when he felt you slide your hand under his coat and fumble with his zipper. What if the cabbie looked back? But as you worked your magic fingers around him, he realized he was getting incredibly hard. You had on a long skirt, and he watched as you maneuvered your panties down one leg, then turned and sat on top of him. He wasn't inside you, but just the touch of flesh on flesh was electric.

When the two of you stumbled out of the cab and walked in the door you ran into the kitchen. He heard you open the refrigerator door and put something on the stove. In a minute, you joined him in the den, wearing only high heels and dangling earrings, carrying a tray. On it was a bottle of massage oil, a bucket of ice cubes, and a pot of warm, steaming honey.

"Lie down for your massage," you ordered.

He went for the blinds, since your apartment was right across from another high-rise, but you stopped his hand. "I want to be seen," you insisted, pushing him down on the rug.

He couldn't wait for his massage. He tested the honey with his finger, and as he knelt before you, he applied it to the creases that run from the tops of your thighs into the hiding place between your legs. It usually took time to arouse you these days, but tonight you were flowing. You dug your fingers into his hair and drew him closer. "I need you inside me," you said.

"Wait." With one hand, he poured the honey down the cleft that led to your clitoris and with the other he took an ice cube and teased your nipples until they were rock hard. Then, before you knew what was happening, he ran the ice down your body and inserted it into your vagina, then bent and hungrily licked a circle around your clitoris, roughly cleaning honey off the shaft and sides with his tongue. You cried out and your body thrashed in his arms, but he held you tight with his mouth, not letting you escape the pleasure.

He wanted you so badly, but to prolong the ecstasy, he rolled you onto your stomach and applied the massage oil down your back and between your legs. The soft, scented essence flowed over you and when he breathed it in it made him ache. He slid across your slick buttocks and added a smaller chip of ice before entering you from behind. You were wild, bucking against him, but he wouldn't let you go. He reached around in front, stimulating you, as his own excitement grew intense.

You began to come again and again, and your face was more beautiful than he'd ever seen it. When he came with you, he wrapped his arms around you. "I love saying goodbye to you," he whispered.

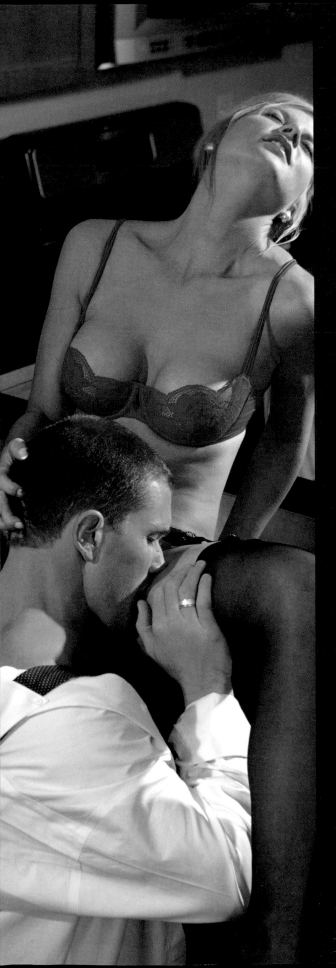

4

Rules of Engagement

NAUGHTY BUT SAFE

A woman turning forty caught my interest when she told me how the scent of flowers becomes her. "We were at a botanical garden, walking through the aisles of the most exotic plants and sensuously scented flowers, and I just couldn't help myself; it was as if I was in a spell. My hand furtively began wandering up and around my husband's groin. He turned and looked at me, our eyes met, we exchanged our most receptive smiles and he became incredibly amorous. It was near closing time so we made our way through the leafy jungle of plants and floral arrangements, and used the deserted, public restroom next to the gardens, and had very fast, very hot sex. It was a celebration of natural beauty and life!"

Another woman a few years older offered this: "By far the best sex my husband and I have had was in a changing room at a department store. Several of the men's changing rooms were being used for storage and we were in hurry, so I talked the clerk into letting us both into the women's changing room. To my husband's surprise I told him to drop his pants and I proceeded to perform oral sex; then I dropped my pants and we had a quickie. It was great—one stop shopping!"

No question, having sex in strange places is a turn-on. We all have a bit of the exhibitionist in us, so the thought of doing something that borders on the forbidden, and the possibility of someone watching, can be exciting.

SEX IN THE BATHROOM

A QUICKIE IN THE BATHROOM, IN FRONT OF THE MIRROR, CAN ADD AN EXCITING, NAUGHTY, AND VOYEURISTIC ASPECT TO YOUR SEX.

The thought of getting caught in the act may also be a turn-on. But that's a thought; it is something to be played with to amp up the excitement. Actually being viewed in public is something else all together.

Outside of the privacy of your own home, having sex in full view is likely to come to the attention of the local authorities. Even if you aren't carted off to sex-crazed prison, it's possible that you will be intruding on someone else's privacy—the "someone" being the person who spots you in a compromising position. No one wants to end up as the opener on the evening news, right?

While the risk of discovery can be highly exciting because it adds a degree of naughtiness, pushing it too far is asking for trouble. Rules are rules. Some are begging to be broken, like "Sshh, no talking in the library," but others, like those concerning lewd behavior, if broken, can have dire consequences.

If we do break rules, most of us do so expecting to get away with it. Some quickies are low-risk, and some border on the compulsive and self-destructive. The trick is to get that thrill in a safe way. Smart people have their moment in the sun in a place and in a manner that is relatively low risk but high return.

That's where it can get a bit complicated. You've heard of opposites attracting. It applies to risk-taking as well. Personality-wise, some of us are more like sheep and some of us more like wolves, and we attract each other.

Sheep are guardians of high standards who dislike having to break the rules. Wolves have fewer problems with violation, feel in control of situations, and exploit opportunities when they arise. Which one are you?

If you're more sheep than wolf, you like continuity and feel comfortable with the familiar. If you're more wolf than sheep, you get bored easily and relish adventure.

A Word to the Wolves

To the wolves among you, keep this in mind: Getting arrested for public indecency is not only going to be embarrassing and costly (fines, litigation, etc.), it is likely to catch the attention of your employer as well. It makes sense to give some thought in advance to your dalliances and scope out your intended rendezvous point for possible problems, interruptions, and routes of escape if necessary.

So how do wolves and sheep pull it off and make it memorable for both of them?

To all you wolves out there, let me start off by emphasizing that I'm all for breaking out of the usual routine but I do not recommend that you let your passion lead you into a situation where you end up having quick sex with someone you don't know or going too far out on a limb with someone you do know. You won't enjoy it, you won't feel good about it, and it could even screw up your health and the way you feel about your sexual encounters in the future.

A Word to the Sheep

You always make love the same way, in the same order of acts, at the same time, and it is satisfying because you know what to expect. At the same time, because you and your partner know what to expect, the sex isn't passionate or sometimes even exciting.

You would be wise to shake things up a bit to revive those feelings of erotic bliss—otherwise your love life may become a strong candidate for the boredom heap. Pushing the

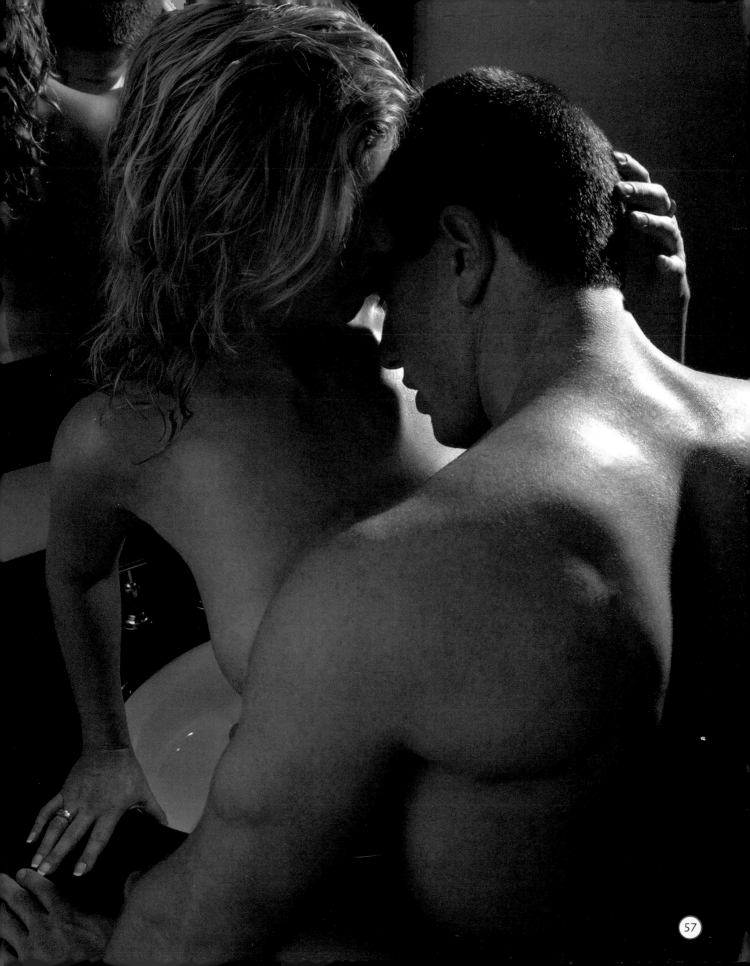

boundaries may be difficult, but there are "safe risks" to consider that combat boredom. These include a naked encounter late at night in your own outdoor pool or hot tub; doing it in the bathroom at a party or restaurant, especially if it's a big city restaurant with the single unisex bathrooms; and performing oral sex upstairs at your parent's house while the family is downstairs putting dinner together. Other possibilities for out-of-the-ordinary locations are private coves on nude beaches, your own office (when you are the boss!), deserted classrooms at a college after hours, or in the middle of the night at (or in) the pool of a hotel where you are a guest and where they have a high tolerance for your privacy.

Sometimes, the adventure doesn't even have to be sexual. There is a basic scientific explanation for that: Sharing new experiences—just taking a challenging, exciting class together—will do it for some couples. New experiences stimulate chemicals in the brain that trigger amorous feelings.

Think back to high school when you watched a horror movie with a guy. He thought you were interested in making out because you grabbed him and fell into his arms at the frightening parts. And there was something to that; you were turned on by the experience of safe fear. We're aroused by fear, which boosts our hormones and sets the stage for stronger emotions and outrageously good sex. A new and shared experience that is challenging can trigger those same feelings.

RULES THAT WORK FOR SHEEP AND WOLVES

Having a set of guidelines that are compatible with wolves as well as sheep will increase the likelihood of having exciting and sexy experiences instead of well-intentioned disasters. Following are the twelve commandments of quickies.

1. **STRANGER DANGER.** Do you know you are safe with the person you're going home with? The excitement of having sex with someone you don't know may be erotic and glamorous, but in reality you must keep yourself safe. Make sure someone knows where you are and whom you are with.

2. **LUBE.** Use a non-oil-based lubrication if you need to. Also, hasty doesn't mean careless; make sure passion and safe sex go hand in hand.

3. **SHH!** Be as quiet as possible. Quickies can be silent, sexual body collisions, and they require a lot more action and a lot less lovey-dovey substance.

4. **BE PRIVATE.** Limit your audience; try to go somewhere as private as possible.

5. **SPEED.** Take heed of why it's called a quickie. The point of a quickie is a speedy release and almost instant gratification. Subtract the unnecessary stuff. Take off as little as possible and keep foreplay (if there's any) to a minimum.

6. **ZIP UP, TUCK IN, AND STRAIGHTEN OUT.** Also be sure to tidy up your hair, as it's usually the number one giveaway that you allowed your inner slut to be free and were engaging in naughty behavior!

7. **STAY AWAY FROM CROWDS.** Seek out reliably secluded spots, such as a remote place to park the car, a deserted beach, an empty, or near-empty movie theater.

8. **SCOPE, WHEN POSSIBLE.** Some places can seem private (such as rooftops) but may not be. It's a good idea to know where you're going and to be familiar with the layout so that you can avoid being seen and avert any possible dangers. When possible, scope out a location first.

9. **HAVE PLAN B READY.** Think about places to duck for cover, ways to camouflage your activity, or a story to tell a possible authority figure. Something better than, "I was minding my own business and he just happened to bump into me."

10. **COMMUNICATE OPENLY.** If you are uncertain about what you want, stop and talk about it. It is okay to be unsure, perhaps that means you want to wait. Remember, if you get crazed about what's happening, you can change your mind. Having said "yes" doesn't mean you can't change your mind. And saying "no" doesn't mean that you won't try something out of the usual routine that is less risky for you.

11. **NO FRILLS, ALL THRILLS.** Forget about candlelight, incense, and seductive music, otherwise all you'll be doing is hyping up an experience that may end up leaving you dissatisfied. The whole point of quickie sex is spontaneity so it's okay if you're in the living room, the TV is on, his pants are down around his ankles, and your skirt is hiked up, way up! That's the beauty of spontaneous, passionate, quickie sex.

12. **DON'T FORGET AURAL SEX.** Not the same as licking and sucking, aural sex involves those little whispers that you and he quietly exchange about how good it feels. Moaning and groaning will flatter him, turn up the heat for both of you, and demonstrate that you're excited about what you're experiencing. Now I'm not suggesting that you fake it, and definitely don't start screaming in a place where you don't want to call attention to yourself, but a little enthusiasm never hurt anyone.

A Note on Safe Sex

If your relationship is monogamous and you are both healthy, safe sex precautions are more about not getting caught being naughty. If your relationship is not monogamous, safe sex precautions are important, not so much about not getting caught, although that is a concern, but more about not getting sick.

If you're not in a monogamous relationship, here are sex activities in ascending order of risk.

Kissing. There is no evidence I am aware of that sexually transmitted diseases (STDs), including HIV, are spread by kissing unless both partners have open sores in their mouths or have bleeding gums. Saliva does not carry the HIV virus. No risk.

Mutual masturbation. No risk as long as your guy does not ejaculate on you.

Erotic massage. No risk in touching and stroking.

Oral sex. Transmission could take place if blood or fluids come in contact with cuts or micro lesions in the mouth or throat. To be completely safe, you should put a condom on your guy for fellatio. Minimal risk.

Vaginal intercourse. STDs (including HIV) can be transmitted this way. Check your partner's genitals for obvious signs of ill health and use condoms. But don't fool yourself into not using a condom if there are no obvious signs of illness on his genitals. More often than not, symptoms don't appear to the eye. Risk activity.

Anal intercourse. Infected semen can easily enter the bloodstream through the membranes of the rectum and through micro tears that may occur during intercourse. If you do have anal intercourse—which I don't recommend with casual partners—use specially designed anal condoms and a lot of water-soluble lubricant. High risk.

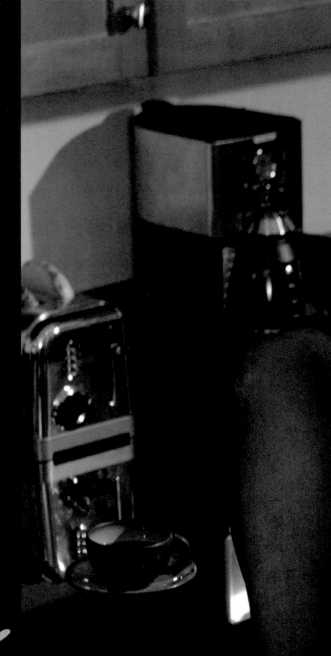

anywhere

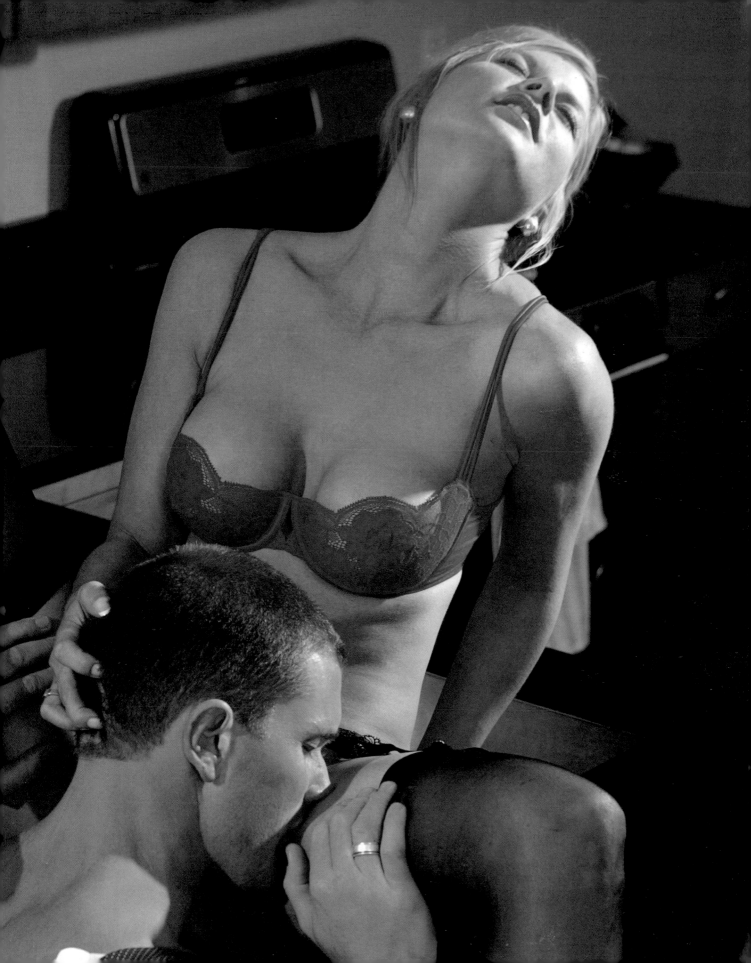

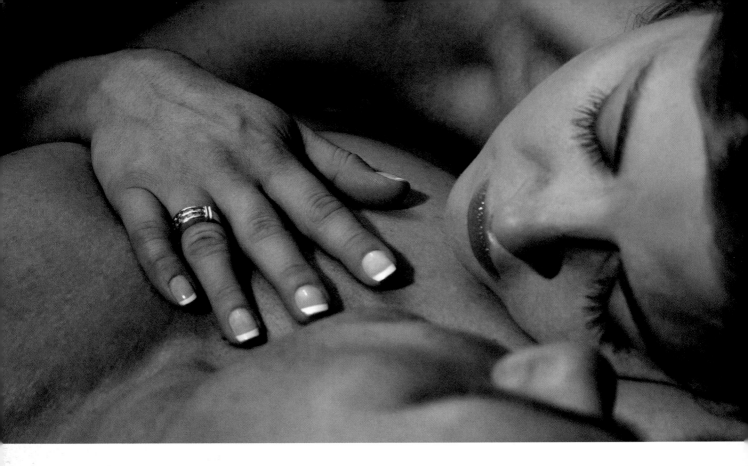

QUICKIE
A SUMPTUOUS
SUNDAY MORNING

You stretch and yawn. The rain is drizzling softly on the windows, drumming a gentle beat that lulls you back to sleep. You can be lazy all day—it's Sunday.

You feel a hand snaking across your warm limbs and it's impossible to ignore. Are you dreaming or waking? Your limbs start to shake in sensuous delight. You can feel a roving mouth and tongue between your legs, and an explosion begins somewhere inside you that you cannot control.

You open your eyes and glance at your lover, whose face bears a silly grin. "Isn't that better than the newspaper and coffee?"

You take your time getting up and dressing, then decide to go out for a drive. The rain has nearly stopped, but everything has a dewy wetness about it. You come to a completely deserted road just off an abandoned highway. It is straight as a pin. "Keep driving," you say, putting one hand on your lover's leg. You begin to stroke it lightly, making circles on his thigh, moving upward an inch at a time. You undo one button, then a zipper, and slip your hand inside. You can feel a quickened pulse under your fingers. There is no one else around—no one else in the world—as you work faster and harder, aiming for delirium. Suddenly, the car jerks to a halt and you are thrown back in your seat. Both of you sit, panting, and then your lover pulls the car over to the side of the road.

You climb into the back seat and loosen each other's clothing. One leg is on the head-rest of the front seat, the other presses against the door latch. Each kiss, each caress, feels like the breeze through the open window. You welcome your lover into your arms, pulling pants in one direction and shirts in another. You lay head to head, trying to accommodate in such close quarters. You feel the pressure of limb on limb as you welcome this wonderful body inside yours.

Monday morning seems as far away as the moon.

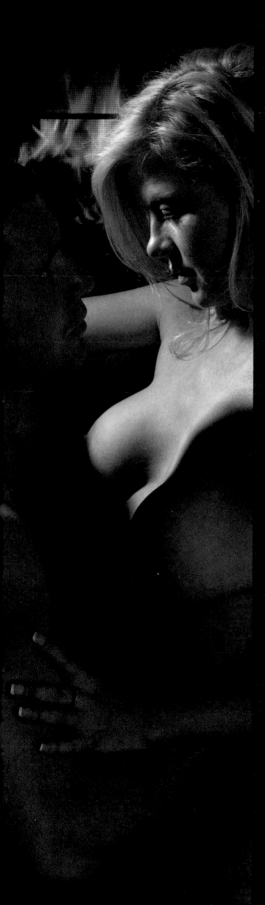

5

Quickie Positions: Location, Location

LIGHTING YOUR FIRE

There are six intercourse positions with each having many possibilities for variation. Some people are restricted to a particular position by pregnancy, obesity, illness, or injury. Habit restricts most others. They may have been experimental early in their relationship, trying a variety of positions, and then they settle into one position and get into the pattern of sameness. If you have intercourse in the same place and in the same position you have always done, it is no wonder why your sex life seems routine and boring. You're overdue for change.

While there are lots of possible variations on the six basic positions, the term "sex positions" takes on a whole new meaning with quickie sex. Often, the usual positions are not practical and couples find themselves in situations that require positions they'd never have otherwise experimented with, particularly because they are not likely to be making love in bed.

Old pieces of furniture, a wall, a throw rug, or anything else that happens to be close by comes into its own when no-frills, all-thrills sex is on the menu. One woman even found a unique use of a washing machine:

"I was folding some clothes and my husband came up behind me and kissed my neck. It felt very sexy and was just the break I needed from the laundry. I turned around and kissed him. We just kept at it, merging into each other, mouth to mouth, breathing as one, tongues flirting, and just taking in marvelous sensations. Next thing I know I am sitting on the washing machine and he is inside me. It all happened so unexpectedly, I felt as if I was playing out a scene in a soft-core movie.

"The freakiest part of this experience was when the spin cycle of the wash started. That put me over-the-top. I went into an orgasmic spin that seemed to last forever! I never got back to the laundry that day; it was as if I spent the rest of the day in an erotic trance. Now when I am doing laundry for two adults and two children the tedium is broken up by a very delicious memory."

Not only are the location and the position different than usual, quickies are usually carried out with one or both partners partially dressed. This in itself can be highly arousing.

The sight of you raising your skirt and bending forward over the kitchen table to reveal your naked thighs and bottom can make even a weary man become fully alert. In equal measure, the feel of his body pressed against yours with your arms held to the wall above your head can bring a rush of energy back into your day.

Being partially or even fully clothed has other sexy advantages. The clothes, to some extent, will get in the way—and that's a good thing. You or your guy may be turned on by the touch or look of certain clothes. The smooth feel of your dress or the sight of you in high heels may make him wild, just as the feel of his clothes against your bare skin can be an exciting bonus of quickie sex for you.

Quickies have other things going for them as well. If your encounter is truly spontaneous you are likely to be unwashed and conse-quently the smell of the day and of your body is going to be more evident. If you have an attitude that is open to this, the earthiness can actually prove to be a real turn-on, as the normal act of washing actually removes many of the naturally occurring chemical scents that can heighten arousal.

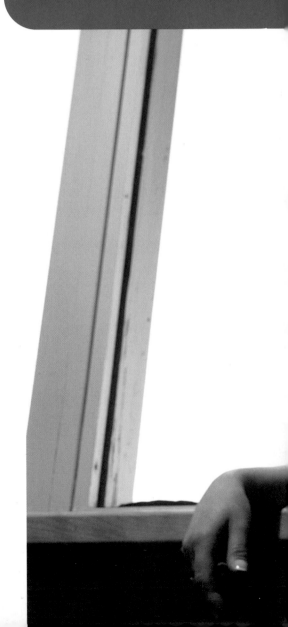

QUICKIE

FULL VIEW

HAVING SEX IN AN ALTERNATIVE LOCATION TO THE BEDROOM IS WHAT QUICKIES ARE ALL ABOUT. THERE ARE PLACES IN YOUR HOME THAT YOU PROBABLY DON'T EVEN REALIZE COULD MAKE A FANTASTIC QUICKIE SPOT, LIKE THIS "ROOM WITH A VIEW."

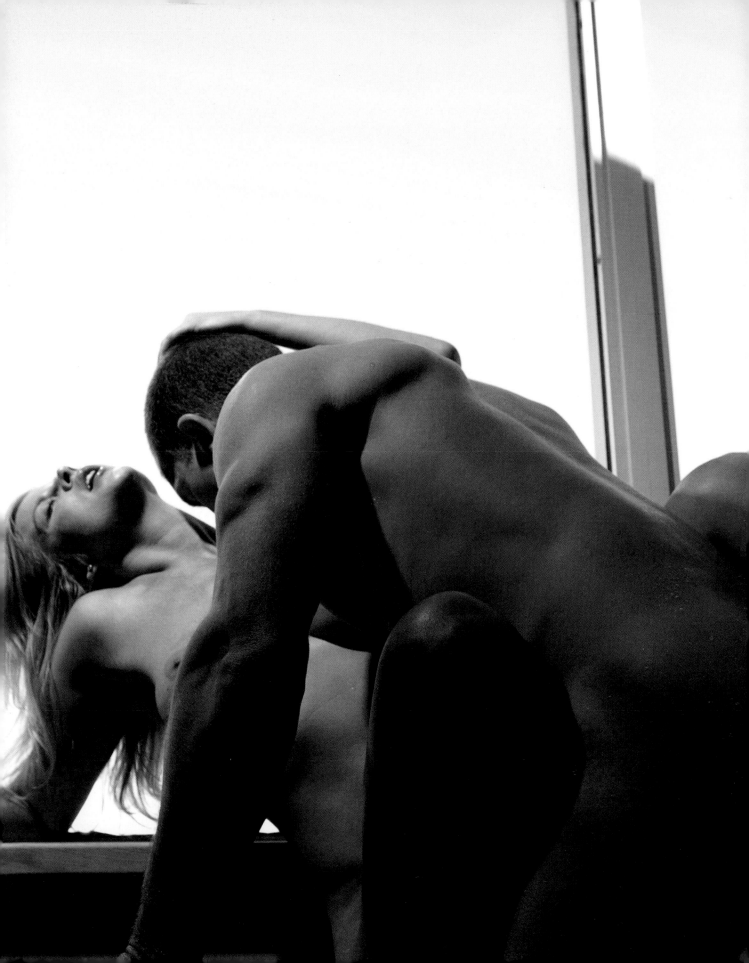

ON THE TOWN

Being in an unconventional location and more spontaneous than the traditional Saturday night encounter in bed has definite benefits. Naughty and unplanned sex can be very hot.

For many people, spontaneous sex is a reminder of the days when they were courting and couldn't get enough of each other, or going back still further in time, living with their parents. The opportunity for physical contact with boyfriends was limited in those days, and most young couples became very innovative at creating moments of intimacy whenever they could.

That's all well and good, but there is a trade-off. While the excitement level is notched up, the comfort level and range of positions isn't going to be as sweet and reliable as your bed. The good news is that I'm betting that it won't matter because the flame is going to be hot enough to compensate.

Even if you're home but not in bed, unfamiliar movements and body positions produce new and stimulating sensations that provide a definite turn-on. But these positions may be a bit awkward for you at first. If you're out on the town, the challenge becomes even greater, as a woman who suggested a late-night poolside romp found out.

"We were in a hotel and it was very late at night. I wasn't quite fully asleep when my boyfriend woke up and started fondling me. I said, 'Let's go down to the pool.' It wasn't as if I had been planning that, the words just spilled from my mouth. We were sleeping naked so we quickly threw on robes and settled into one of the chairs by the edge of the pool. It was completely deserted at this hour. I lay on the chair on my stomach and he got on top of me, positioning his legs on either side of mine. As he entered me, I closed my legs and crossed them at the ankles.

"With my legs clenched and ankles crossed, I was able to feel the entire length of him inside me and grip it tight, creating loads of feel-good friction. He was also able to reach under me and play with my nipples, which are very sensitive. Things were going really well, I was right there about to come when suddenly the chair tipped. I hadn't realized how much we were rocking. We both landed in the water, which dampened my orgasm—and his—especially since he doesn't swim!"

Anytime, anyplace can be great fun and extraordinarily sexy, but unless you're a masochist, you'll want to take some precautions. For example, if you're romping in an alley or on the side of the road—such as the couple whose car was too small for the romp, but big enough to block the roadside view— you'll want minimal contact with concrete.

In the outdoor concrete jungle you'll want to avoid road rash, keep your clothes from getting dirty, and protect your bottom from freezing over. And, depending where you are, on a staircase for example, you'll want to avoid taking a tumble. It almost goes without saying that in many of these situations your best bet is to be in an inconspicuous position so that it's not obvious to anyone who might catch you in the act.

Assuming the Position

Quickies in semi-public places—in woods, fields, or even your own backyard—heighten your arousal through the sense of naughtiness you experience. But, if you're not looking to make the next day's news headline or be the graphic feature on someone's cell phone, consider a position convenient for leaving your clothes on whilst engaging in the act. Let's say you're on a park bench and no one is around. You just finished having lunch and you both are in the "lust is a must" mode.

If you're wearing a long skirt, you can sit on his lap facing him with your legs underneath you on the bench. Let your skirt drape over you, and put your arms on his shoulders for balance as he brings one hand under your skirt and finds a home between your legs. Get to work gliding up and down as unobtrusively as possible. This position is hot, much easier than squatting, and almost discreet.

A slight variation for that roadside or alleyway quickie: He squats on his heels while you sit on his upper thighs facing him with your weight on your feet. Wrap your arms around him for balance—or, one arm around him and the other down between your legs to provide some additional clit friction, if needed.

Another position, standing and facing each other, is very intimate and sexy; it is a favorite of the quickie set. This type of encounter will work well on staircases in an office building, in your apartment house (or his), or any other place where you can easily adjust for height differences.

Aside from adjusting for height differences, someplace where the playing field is *not* level affords you the opportunity to lift one leg (for example, like on a toilet seat) for easier entry. If there is a significant height difference and your guy can lift and hold you with your legs wrapped around him, you needn't go on a hunt for a hidden staircase; standing and facing each other will work down a dark alley, in a hidden corner of a large library, and other such forbidden places. Once again, for easy access, wear that easy-to-lift skirt that you've been saving for the occasion.

What if there is a height difference and he isn't going to be able to suspend you long enough to get rockin'? I've got a remedy for that. Come on, you knew this one was coming. In fact, many women enjoy this position very much because it allows the man to penetrate them fully.

Here's how it goes: Put your hands on a chair, desk, couch, or wall, and lean forward with your butt into the air. Your guy penetrates you from behind. You will need to tilt your pelvic region to ease his entry into your vagina. He's going to control the frequency of the thrusting.

Another position, standing and facing each other, is very intimate and sexy; it is a favorite of the quickie set.

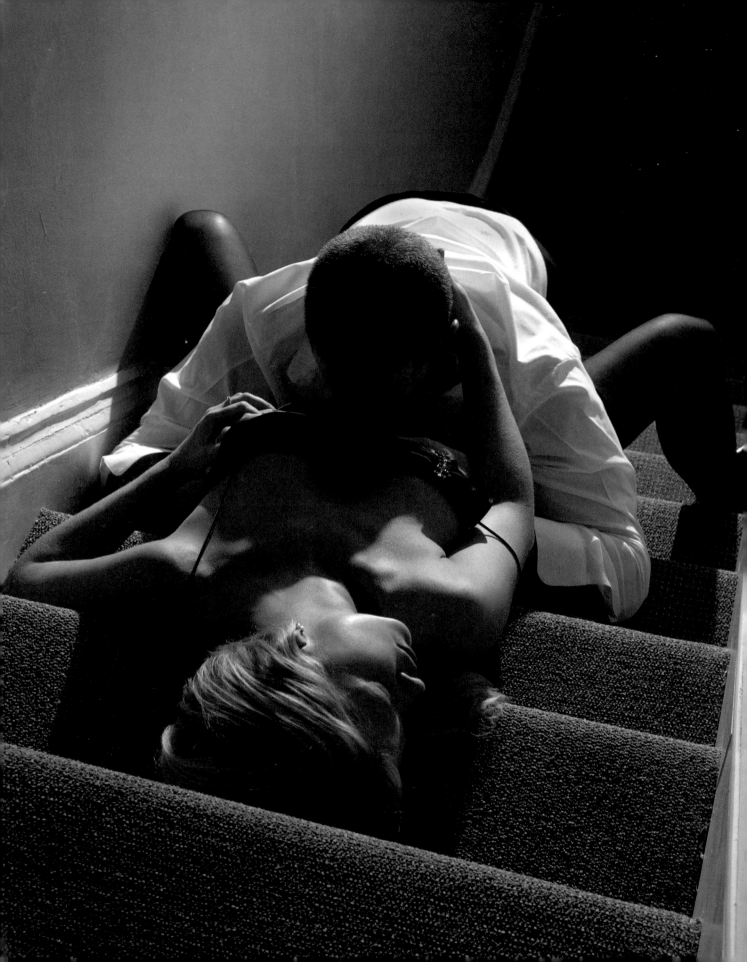

STAIRWAY INTERLUDE

YOU CAN TAKE YOUR SEX UP A NOTCH WITH A QUICKIE STAIRWAY INTERLUDE. THE DIFFERENCE IN HEIGHT AND LEVEL THAT THE STAIRS PROVIDE WILL ALLOW FOR A VARIETY OF INTERESTING POSITIONS.

To help steady himself, he can hold onto your butt/hips and thrust. In an unconventional location, flirting with the forbidden, couples often enjoy hard thrusting. This position is much easier to achieve than the standard face-to-face position and it affords him the freedom to massage your breasts, and to reach down and manually stimulate your clitoris with his hand—or for you to do so.

In a slight variation, go lower. Bend forward as low as you are comfortable with, your legs slightly spread and your arms either hanging loose in front of you or resting on a low chair for balance. Your guy enters you from behind, pulling himself as close to you as possible while holding your torso for support.

This scorching little spin on rear-entry is perfect for I-need-you-now quickies. Bending over really low gives your guy maximum depth and control, and if you are sensitive in this area, the angle allows good access to your G-spot. Unlike typical rear-entry action that can leave you feeling disconnected from your guy, your pelvises and thighs touch, making the move more intimate.

Want a little control? Urge him to stay still while you grind your behind in circles. And don't forget to add that extra zing— either you or he can reach between your legs to attend to your C-spot.

If your height affords a really good fit with your guy, have him stand in front of you with your legs spread wide apart so that he can plunge deep inside. If you're sufficiently aroused before this occurs—and you better be, or else you're not ready and should tell him so—it's sure to cause you to reach climax quickly. Once again, in a new and daring location, it may be easier and quicker for you to get aroused than you realize.

It is often said that good sex depends on meticulous foreplay to arouse the woman so that her vagina is lubricated. That's often true for routine, conventional sex, but your vagina can lubricate almost immediately when you are in the mood for quick sex. In fact, many women are more turned on by quickie sex not only because of the novelty and naughtiness of it, but because of the intense degree of passionate feelings involved.

Whatever position you get into during quickie sex, focus on your pleasure, not on the technical aspects of the position or if you are feeling a bit embarrassed. Don't focus on a nagging guilt about your guy doing more work, or concern over whether he is being pleasured. It may be desirable to communicate about such things, but the focus should be on your sensations and pleasure.

POSITION BASICS

Sometimes you need more than a few minutes, a penis, a vagina, and a connection for a quickie. What's really important is how you feel about the position.

If you feel restrained—I'm not talking hand-cuffs here, I'm referring to *unwanted* restraint of movement—or feel less stimulation in a certain position, you're going to be unhappy and less likely to enjoy yourself. In which case, no amount of adjustment, repositioning, or stimulation will work.

Sure, visualizing sexy positions is fun and arousing, but ask yourself these four key questions so that you can avoid the chiropractor (unless he's your guy!) and get the most bang for your romp.

1. Can you comfortably get in the position and hold it easily enough?
2. Is this position conducive for orgasm? The setting is different, but are you getting clitoral stimulation by him or from yourself?
3. Is the position visually stimulating to you and your partner without being embarrassing to you?
4. Do you have the freedom of movement that is comfortable for you?

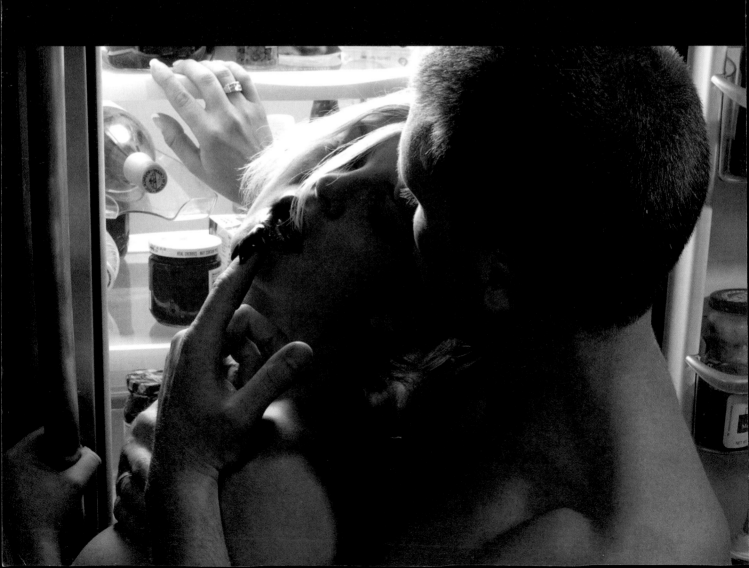

QUICKIE
THE LOVE BANQUET

You've put together a recipe for some mouth-watering lovemaking: Special treats are on hand for when you feel hungry for each other. There's whipped cream, smooth peanut butter, bananas, chocolate sauce, and maple syrup. If you aren't yet mutually monogamous, you'll use fresh fruit, honey, jellies, syrups, or powdered sugar—these won't damage a latex condom. You're planning to apply these foods to your delicious bodies and nibble, suck, lick, and chew them off.

You may want to have your love banquet right in the kitchen, because it's going to be messy. If the counter is long enough, remove the toaster and the food processor and put down a few towels. If you'd prefer a softer surface, strip your bed and use an old sheet. If the weather's good and you have a patio with some privacy, you may decide on a picnic outside.

Eating food off each other will sensitize your taste buds, your tongue, and your mouth. When you lick food and skin at the same time, you'll get a whole different flavor. You have to be very gentle, especially around the vulva and clitoris, and around the penis and testicles. But you'll find, as you consume and caress at the same time, that your awareness is heightened. Your senses of taste, smell, sight, and touch will all be intensified.

He starts with an appetizer, a nicely mashed avocado. Using his fingers, he puts a dollop of bright green fruit on your belly. Then, using a chip, he swipes some guacamole and puts it in your mouth. Then he feeds himself, right from the source. His lips scour your stomach—he enjoys the way you moan as he grazes.

To clear his palate, he takes a fresh orange and squeezes it over your breasts. He laps the juice from your nipples, and then you both squeeze what's left in the orange right into each other's mouths.

The main course comes in two parts. First he takes a spray canister of whipped cream and shoots a dab between your legs. He licks and sucks up the cream as you pay attention to every sensation. Not biting but gently nipping, you feel like you are going to scream, and you do.

He looks up at you with a mischievous smile. Slowly, deliberately, he plants a swipe of peanut butter between your legs and dribbles smooth melted chocolate over his penis. He positions himself so that you can (very carefully!) lick the chocolate while he goes in search of the peanut butter.

Don't count calories! You'll work off what you consume and more as soon as you take a shower and throw yourselves into each other, your sexual appetites aroused but not nearly sated.

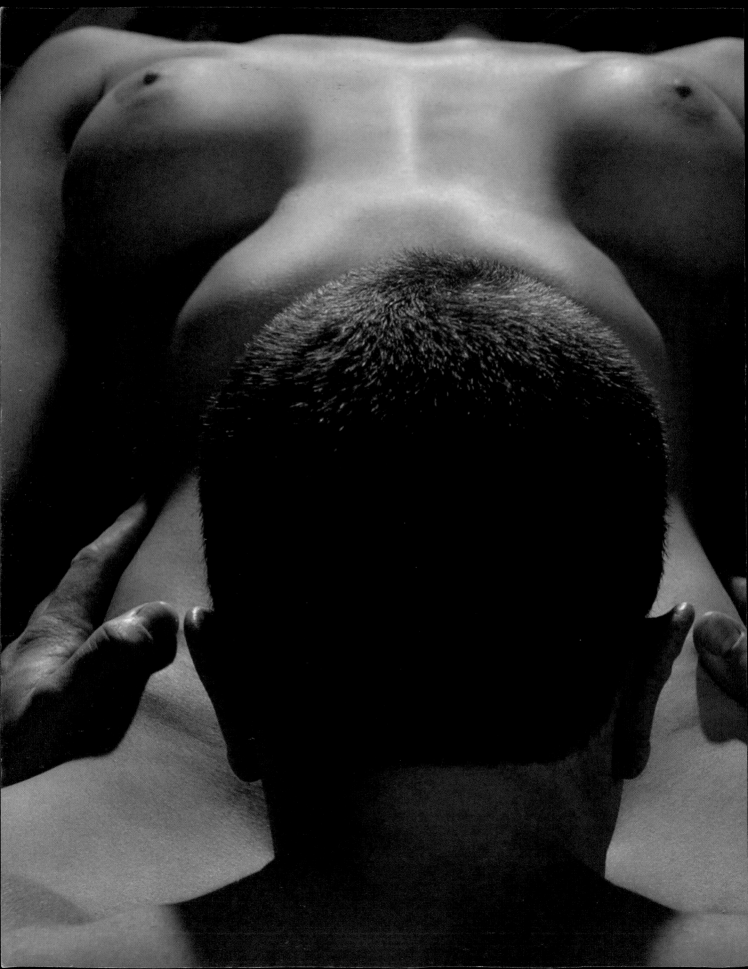

PART TWO:

The Quickie orgasm

HURRY-UP HELPERS

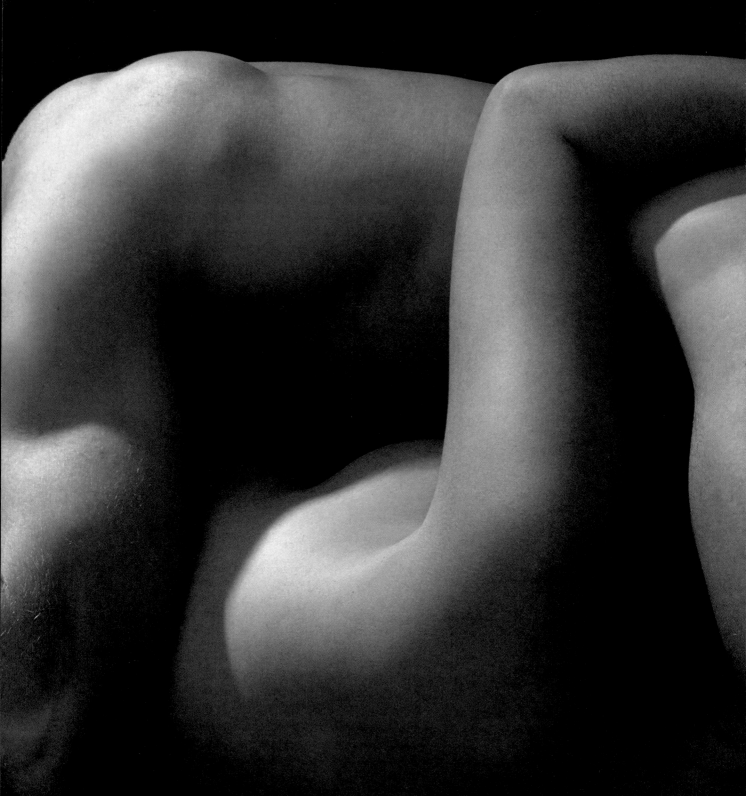

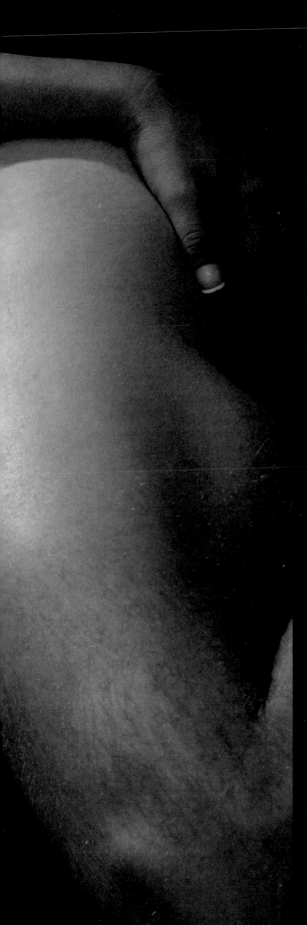

6

The Quickie Orgasm:
Going Downtown

THE ORGASM QUIZ

Welcome to the first part of a three-step process for making orgasm easier and faster. The French call orgasm *le petit mort*, the little death. The roots of the word "orgasm" come from the Greek *orgasmus*, meaning to grow ripe, swell, and be lustful. Romance novelists describe it in "earth-moving" terms.

Poetry and aesthetics aside, an orgasm is a series of rhythmic contractions typically lasting three to twenty seconds, with intervals of less than a second between the first three to six contractions. The contractions are felt in the vagina, anal sphincter, and uterus.

Some women continue to experience these genital spasms for a minute or longer. In fact, some women report post-orgasmic contractions, particularly in the uterus, up to twenty-four hours later. After orgasm, the blood that has concentrated in the area makes a slower trip back to the rest of the body than it does in men, which partially explains why women can reach orgasm and experience orgasm again more quickly than men do.

Orgasm is third in the four stages of sexual excitement observed by renowned sex researchers Masters and Johnson: desire, arousal, orgasm, and resolution. During arousal, as orgasm approaches, blood flow increases to the vagina causing lubrication and swelling of the inner and outer lips and the clitoris.

You know what you want—an orgasm that is reliable, brings release, and is easy and fun. But what's your orgasmic experience now?

The questions below will help you establish your starting point. This is not a test, and there are no right or wrong answers.

1. List all the ways you become orgasmic, including oral sex, masturbation, manual stimulation by your partner, intercourse, or other means.
2. Do you experience orgasm differently, depending on the way it was achieved? Can you explain the differences?
3. How frequently do you reach orgasm during lovemaking?
4. Have you ever had or do you sometimes or often have multiple orgasms?
5. Have you ever experienced an extragenital orgasm, that is, an orgasm achieved with stimulation to areas other than the genitals?
6. Have you ever felt an orgasm in parts of your body other than the genitals?
7. Be as specific as possible in describing exactly what kinds of stimulation, including pressure and amount, bring you to orgasm.
8. How do your emotions and feelings toward your partner affect your orgasms?
9. How do your partner's orgasms affect yours?
10. Do you have a particularly sensitive body part (aside from the genitals) that, when stimulated at the same time your genitals are being stimulated, affects orgasm?

Orgasm is a blend of physical, psychological, and emotional factors. The orgasmic experience varies depending on the type of sexual activity, the closeness felt toward your partner, and other conditions. Your answers to the ten questions above will help you develop a better awareness of how you reach orgasm, differentiate the feelings of orgasms achieved using different methods of stimulation, and assess how much you may have been limiting orgasmic potential by attitudes and behaviors.

I believe that you can experience orgasm more fully and faster than you do now. What can stop you? Two things: thinking that you can't and using exactly the same approach to reach orgasm as you do now. It's time for a sexual shake-up.

CLIT POWER

Although the G-spot gets a lot of attention for being your erotic epicenter, it's the clitoris that packs the most pleasurable punch for you during sex. In the majority of women the clitoris is the most sensitive area of their genitals. There are more nerve endings in the C-spot than there are in any other erotic area of your entire body.

A button-sized organ located just below the place where the tops of the inner labia meet, the head of the clitoris is often partially or totally hidden by the clitoral hood, a fold of skin. The shaft is largely covered by the labia and extends inside the body into the pubic region.

The clitoris is highly sensitive to stimulation. As a woman becomes aroused by clitoral stimulation or other means, the organ pulls back against the pubic bone and the labia swell, making the clitoris appear erect. This is why it is sometimes compared to the penis.

Because of its small size and hidden location, the clitoris has been—and to some extent remains—shrouded in mystery. Men often report trouble in locating it or confusion about how and when to stimulate it. In fact, as nearly every woman will attest, when it comes to understanding female sexuality, most guys know more about what's under the hood of a car than under the hood of a clitoris. Though less than a third of women reach orgasm through intercourse without clitoral stimulation, many women are shy about asking for it and afraid of intimidating or belittling their partner by touching themselves during lovemaking. And while it seems that men have struggled valiantly since the dawn of time to find ways to reliably elicit the female orgasm, rare is the guy who has the modesty to ask, "What can I do?"

Compounding the problem, theories about how women *should* be orgasmic have come in and out of fashion over the years, with some schools of thought, most notably Freud's, maintaining the superiority of vaginal or non-clitoral orgasms. This kind of thinking has done a great deal of harm to women and to their relationships with men.

The clitoris is the key to orgasm, and in nearly all women it is a source of pleasure that should not be overlooked. In fact, it is, for the vast majority of women, as close to a magic button as can be found. Here's what a sampling of women say about the clitoris.

From a forty-one-year-old woman married thirteen years: "I've never had an orgasm through intercourse. I met Frank when I was twenty-eight and had been sexually active for nearly ten years. There were lots of lovers before him, with different techniques and different staying power, but I didn't have an orgasm with any of them. After Frank and I were married a while, we had established enough trust and comfort with each other to talk about and work out the right kind of clitoral stimulation to make me orgasmic."

A twenty-seven-year-old woman who does not have a steady partner says: "I've never had a vaginal orgasm, an orgasm that didn't include direct clitoral stimulation. I feel most confident that I will be orgasmic if I stimulate myself because I need specific rhythm and pressure. Sometimes a lover can do it, especially with his tongue, which I find very hot! When I have intercourse I prefer positions that allow me to touch my clitoris. That way I can have an orgasm during intercourse and really enjoy it!"

From a thirty-three-year-old divorced woman: "I am easily orgasmic, which I am sure has more to do with luck than anything else. I can have orgasms during intercourse without direct clitoral stimulation. But sometimes I prefer to touch myself during intercourse and come that way. The orgasm is faster and feels stronger, as if it were coming from several places at once."

Because of its small size and hidden location, the clitoris has been—and to some extent remains—shrouded in mystery. Men often report trouble in locating it or confusion about how and when to stimulate it.

FINGER POWER

Want to speed up your sexual response? More than any other activity, masturbation is the most important activity to quicken your orgasm. Some years ago, Diane Grosskopf was commissioned by *Playgirl* to study 1,207 women. Okay, *Playgirl* isn't exactly a scientific journal, but the results were so clear-cut it's hard to dismiss.

Masturbation was shown to produce orgasm more reliably than any other source of stimulation. It turns out the culturally ingrained symbol of manhood, the penis, is not the ultimate sexual magic wand.

It comes down to this: Get your C-spot used to a quick response by practicing—letting your hand show you the way. Issues such as inexperience, inhibition, and fear can slow or even cheat you out of having an orgasm, but the most common issue is something so simple it is not given enough thought—friction directed to the clitoris. As we'll see in the pages that follow, regardless of how friction is applied, your orgasm is almost always the result of clitoral stimulation.

Research reveals that the more orgasms you have, the more easily you'll have orgasms. So the rumors you've heard are true: Women who regularly let their fingers do the walking require less time to become aroused, and experience more orgasms, increased sexual desire, and greater relationship satisfaction.

In addition, women who masturbate learn to concentrate on their own feelings during sex. Most women are too concerned with pleasing their partners or worried about their failure to reach orgasm, which is a major distraction that masturbation can help alleviate. **Bottom line: Masturbation is essential and is the first step in your three-phase effort to become more easily orgasmic.**

Follow these steps to initiate the process of becoming more orgasmic, or if you've already started, to speed your progress.

1. **BEGIN IN A RELAXED STATE.** Take a warm bath or have a glass of wine. Ensure your privacy and avoid distractions: Turn off all the phones, lock the door, and if the kids are around make sure they are occupied and that you will not be disturbed. If your children are very young, wait until they are asleep or for a time when you have someone to look after them. Find a comfy position. Most women start out lying on their backs, legs bent and spread apart, with feet on the ground. Remove most or all of your clothing.

2. **FANTASIZE.** Recall an exciting past sexual encounter or elaborate on a favorite sexual fantasy. If you need a boost, look at a sexy magazine, read an erotic story, or watch an adult video. Give yourself permission to explore these images in your mind—anything goes as long as it heightens your excitement. There are no thought police!

3. **BE SENSUAL.** For the moment, think of yourself as blind and run your hands along parts of your body to visualize what you look like. Linger along areas that are more responsive to touch than others. Look at your genitals in a mirror (especially if you're unfamiliar with them) and caress the different parts to see what feels especially good. Find and touch your inner and outer labia, your clitoris, your vagina, and your perineum—the area between the vagina and the anus.

4. **TOUCH.** Using one or two fingers, rhythmically stroke the different parts of your vulva, paying particular attention to your clitoris and labia. Experiment with different types of pressure, speed, and motion. Try placing a finger on either side of the clitoris and stroking up and down, or placing two fingers on the clitoral hood and rubbing in a circular motion.

5. **EXPLORE.** Bear in mind that each person's genitals are unique and your method of creating pleasure with your genitals may not be exactly at the same pace or with the same touch as someone else. That doesn't matter, as long as you are able to bring your stroking technique into the lovemaking with your partner. Try different types and rate of touch; explore a lighter, faster stroke, a firmer, slower stroke and any combination that feels good. For some women the best stroke is one that moves around the clitoris rather than the one that applies direct pressure.

6. **TEASE.** Build up your sexual excitement and hold on to it before backing off a bit by reducing or temporarily stopping the stimulation. The beauty of this roller-coaster method is that arousal mounts to such intensity that when you finally let yourself go, you're practically guaranteed an outrageous orgasm. Pay attention to how your body is responding. It will tell you the particular stroke that feels best and when to pick up or slow down the tempo.

7. **BREATHE.** Focusing on your breathing is probably the last thing you want to think about when you're being sexual, but your breathing pattern can help increase an orgasm's impact. Don't hold your breath; breathe deeply but rapidly as your arousal builds to help release the sexual energy rather than fight it.

    As you feel the orgasm approach, try breathing more strongly and consciously than usual. You'll increase the tension through your whole abdomen and upper body, raising the intensity of your ecstasy. As you do this, rhythmically clench and release your PC muscle (see the sidebar, page 83, for specific directions on how to clench your pelvic floor muscles).

As nearly every woman will attest, when it comes to understanding female sexuality, most guys know more about what's under the hood of a car than under the hood of a clitoris.

8. **GET OVER THE TOP.** If your hand gets tired, give yourself a rest, switch hands, or try a vibrator. If you're on the brink of orgasm but can't quite get over, amp up your fantasy by imagining a really hot movie. (More will be said about this when we get to step two in the following chapter.) You may also give yourself extra stimulation by caressing other hot spots on your body: your nipples, perineum, or any other spot you've discovered to be a turn-on.

9. **RIDE THE WAVE.** As you begin to orgasm, continue the stimulation through the orgasm. Lighten up on the stimulation during the first extremely sensitive moments but keep it going to enjoy those pleasurable aftershocks. Your first orgasm may feel like a blip or a blast, but the more you practice, the more variety you will experience.

10. **PERSIST.** Didn't work? Don't get discouraged, visualize being successful and with continued practice you will be. Research suggests a positive attitude about your responsiveness will help your body become more responsive. You may also want to try some of the following helpers:

Vibrators take some of the manual labor out of masturbation by providing direct, intense physical stimulation to the clitoris.

Water helps many women learn to masturbate. Lie back in a bath tub with your legs spread and direct the stream of water from the shower head at your clitoris.

Vary the pressure, the pulsation, and the temperature. Want something more upscale? Use Jacuzzi jets.

Dildos can be pleasurable accompaniments to clitoral masturbation, as they offer the fullness of penetration and can also stimulate the G-spot.

If you start making love more often, even if it's a little pleasure date with yourself, the better you will become at it and the more you will enjoy it. It's a chemical thing—the communication between brain cells quickens and intensifies because the impulses are traveling a well-defined, familiar path. It's like other physical activities, practice makes the effort more efficient.

Here are a few additional tips.

1. Studies have shown that erotic highs from masturbation can last several hours. Speed things up by letting your fingers do the walking long before your guy is on the scene. What if the mood is there, but he isn't? You've had a little pleasure date with yourself, and what's wrong with that?

If you want to wait until he's on the scene, that approach works too. In one poll, 95 percent of men said it's a major turn-on watching his lover please herself. Besides, it takes some of the pressure off him.

2. Touching the clitoris directly may be too intense for some women, which means that instead of building up arousal you may feel discomfort. To avoid this, press your index finger and middle fingers on either side of your outer lips, gently squeezing your fingers together in a circular motion to stimulate the clitoral ridge underneath.

3. When he shows up, stay self-interested. If you focus on pleasing him—Is he enjoying this? Is he into me?—you'll distract yourself and cut down on your own pleasure. Keep in mind that the best thing you can do for him is to allow your own pleasure to flow.

THE JOY OF MUTUAL MASTURBATION

When you've become comfortable and skilled at bringing yourself to orgasm, consider inviting your guy to be part of the experience as this woman did.

"Ryan wasn't in the mood for sex one night, so I asked him if he would mind if I masturbated in bed," Jessica told me. She and Ryan, both in their forties, have been lovers for seven years. "He feigned nonchalance, but I could tell he was intrigued," she said. "I'd wanted to do this for years, but I was afraid I'd look funny or be too self-conscious to have an orgasm while he was watching. Suddenly my inhibitions were gone. I wanted to show off. I was confident in my ability to have an orgasm any time I wanted one.

"I sat up with my back against the head-board, my legs open, bent up at the knees. First, I massaged my nipples slowly with the flat of my hands. I took each nipple between my fingers and twisted gently, then massaged with my fingers. Moving my hands down toward my genitals at a leisurely pace, I caressed my body. By the time I parted my lips and placed two fingers in V position alongside my clitoris, Ryan was watching me with glazed eyes.

"'Touch your penis,' I told him; he obeyed me in an erotic trance. We masturbated to climax, watching each other, watching ourselves, catching glimpses in the dresser mirror. It was an intensely erotic experience that energized us for days afterward."

Many women find the idea of masturbating in front of their partner unappealing or intimidating. They think masturbation should be private or that couples shouldn't masturbate at all. Many men rate watching a woman masturbate at the top of their sex wish list.

"We masturbated to climax, watching each other, watching ourselves, catching glimpses in the dresser mirror. It was an intensely erotic experience that energized us for days."

Why masturbate together?

> Watching one another fondle genitals from a slight distance is a unique, intensely arousing experience.

> Each partner's excitement feeds the other's, creating a higher level of arousal than either would experience masturbating alone.

> The gift of masturbation increases intimacy between partners.

> It allows both partners to explore their own bodies at their own pace while being stimulated by their lover's presence.

> There's no clearer way to show a partner how you would like to be touched. If your needs have changed and your partner's lovemaking hasn't, play a little show rather than tell.

> It's a great inhibition-breaker for stimulating yourself during intercourse with your partner.

For more variety, introduce the vibrator, first using it on yourself during masturbation and gradually adding it, on occasion, to your intercourse encounters.

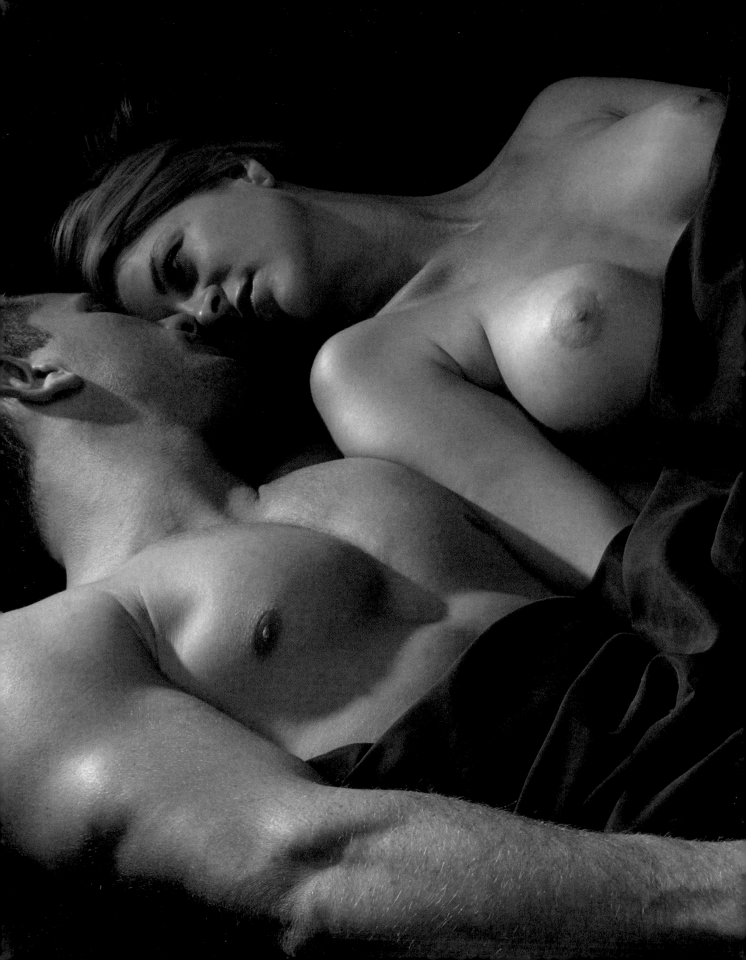

MUTUAL MASTURBATION

WATCHING YOUR LOVER AS YOU MUTUALLY MASTURBATE CAN BE AN INTENSELY EROTIC EXPERIENCE. EACH PARTNER'S EXCITEMENT FEEDS THE OTHER'S, CREATING A HIGHER LEVEL OF AROUSAL THAN ONE MIGHT EXPERIENCE ALONE.

VULVA PUSH-UPS

Use the following technique to make your orgasms longer, stronger, more intense, and just plain better.

The pubococcygeal (PC) muscle group, which supports the pelvic floor, is the one that spasms when you have an orgasm. The clitoris rests on these muscles, so if it's in good shape, more blood will flow to the pelvic area during arousal and the PC will contract more strongly, making orgasms last longer and feel more intense.

The following exercise, called Kegels, after the physician who first suggested it, is a simple way to strengthen PC muscles. No one will know what you're doing, so go ahead and squeeze when your boss is carrying on about this year's goals.

> Squeeze the muscle you use to voluntarily hold back your urine.
> Hold it for two seconds and then release.
> Repeat twenty times, three times a day.

Tip: Perform this exercise during intercourse, squeezing as he slides out and releasing as he plunges in. It'll create tantalizing tension for both of you.

Touch

QUICKIE
HOTEL ADVENTURE

He makes reservations, but doesn't tell you. Instead, you agree to meet him in the hotel bar for a drink after work. When you walk in and ask for him, the mâitre d' hands you a note with a key to the room. The note says, "This key will open the door to an erotic evening you won't want to miss. Follow your heart upstairs."

The room is dark as you enter. He comes up behind you and takes you around the waist, kissing you from behind. The adult channel is playing on the TV screen across the room, and you catch a glimpse of two naked people playfully chasing each other across a tennis court. It's funny and sexy at the same time.

He takes some silk scarves out of his pocket and ties your hands behind your back. Then he takes another scarf and covers your eyes, whispering that he has a wonderful surprise for you. He opens the bottle of wine he's ordered from room service, and you can hear the pop of the cork. He pulls off the coverlet and turns down the sheets—you can hear his hand gliding across the smooth cotton and imagine his fingers doing the same to you.

He guides you into the bathroom where he has already turned on the heating lamp. The room is toasty, and as he begins to touch you softly through your clothes, you can feel how excited he is. He removes your shoes and then, kneeling before you, reaching under your skirt, he teasingly pulls down your panties. He kisses your stomach and thighs, listening to you moan softly.

He opens the sample bottle of body lotion on the counter and massages all your crevices, from your toes to your waist. When you are thoroughly lubricated, he takes his hands off you, leaving you in a state of high desire, telling you how exciting he finds making love to you away from home.

He guides you to the bed and holds the glass of wine so that you can sip from it. If it spills, so much the better—he licks off the excess. He removes the blindfold so that you can take the rest of your clothes off and his too.

For a while, you lie together watching the onscreen couple getting it on. The rhythm of their movements is too tantalizing to ignore, and soon the two of you are locked together, ignoring everything in the world except the sound of your beating hearts and quickened breath.

Now it's his turn to wear the blindfold. Amazing how each touch of your hand and mouth is heightened when he can't see.

"What would you like me to do to you?" you ask.

"Never stop touching me," he tells you ardently. You slide down and take his penis into your mouth as the room spins wildly.

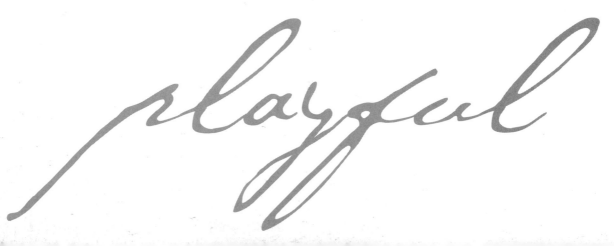

playful

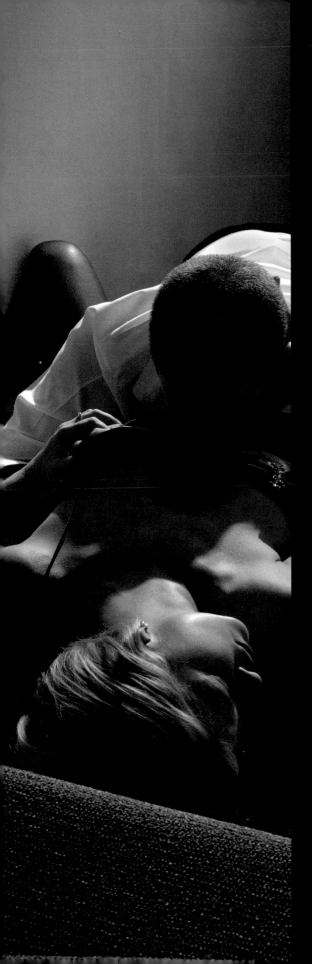

7

The Quickie Orgasm: Brain Sex

WATCHING THE MOVIE IN YOUR HEAD

What if you find yourself making a mental grocery list mid-act? Not likely if you're having sex in the park, but it brings up a point: If you get distracted during sex, your orgasm is down for the count. And it's not necessarily about the distraction of stress.

There is evidence to demonstrate that positive anxiety (for example, as a result of a daring sexual encounter) can increase sexual arousal by concentrating the mind. It works in the same way that being on the edge of danger alerts and heightens all your senses.

So, if you're in a quickie location that has your mind screaming *Wow!* you may not need to show a sexy movie in your head. But short of that, erotic thoughts are essential.

Fantasies often have been compared to private movies running in the theater of our mind. Researchers believe that sexual fantasy is a nearly universal experience among women as well as men, with some of these erotic day-dreams being nothing more than fleeting thoughts like the clips of coming attractions, while others are full-blown features.

A man may glimpse a flash of thigh in a restaurant when a woman crosses her legs and briefly imagine her naked with those legs wrapped around him. A woman may light candles in her bedroom, put on some jazz, and mas-turbate while fantasizing about being taken by her carpen-ter. Each is having a sexual fantasy.

The tangled roots of fantasy lie in childhood. Dr. John Money, one of the world's leading researchers in human sexuality and the pioneer in studying the origins of sexual fantasies, contends they originate before ,puberty, between the ages of five and eight, and then emerge in adolescence.

The child who played at his mother's feet may become the teenager fantasizing about a cheerleader's legs, and eventually become the adult who proudly refers to himself as a "leg" man. Beautiful female legs will likely play a featured role in his fantasies throughout his life.

Some fantasies, like those involving less mainstream practices, such as spanking, fetishes, or bondage, may have less obvious origins, but Money believes their roots can be traced to childhood events as well. A little boy who gets an erection when spanked or a little girl who becomes aroused during a spanking, for example, may, as adults, have spanking fantasies that they don't necessarily want to act out. The awesome power of erotic fantasies comes   from these deep roots embedded in the adult psyche.

Our favorite internally triggered fantasies probably attain preferred status through classical conditioning, the same process that had Pavlov's dogs drooling at the sound of a bell. Fantasies that accompany orgasms are particularly reinforced, for instance, making them more arousing the next time around. From there we embellish and change our fantasies. They're like an evolving series. Scenarios that don't accompany arousal are discarded.

Many people have favored fantasies, those scenarios that can arouse them over and over again. Fantasies, whether violent or repetitive, are a concern only if they inhibit, rather than enhance, sexual expression, and most fantasies don't. In fact, what we know about fantasies is proof enough that they are an important part of our sexual repertoire.

Far from being a sign of sexual inadequacy or deprivation, fantasies are associated with

WHETHER THIS IS IN PLACE OF A QUICKIE, OR A PRELUDE OF ONE TO COME, BOTH PARTNERS ARE GUARANTEED TO EXPERIENCE PLEASURE.

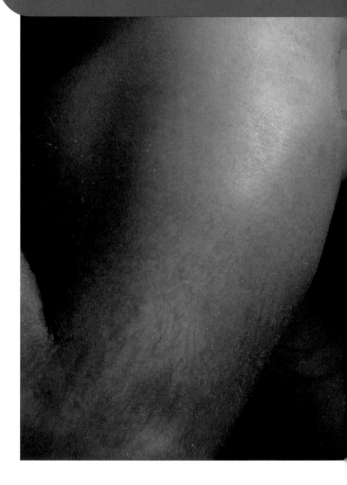

a healthy, happy sex life. Women who have the most sexual problems fantasize the least, and those who reach orgasm easily give their imagination free rein. The three most common fantasies women have include the following:

1. Novel or "forbidden" imagery. This includes unconventional settings, questionable partners like strangers or rela-

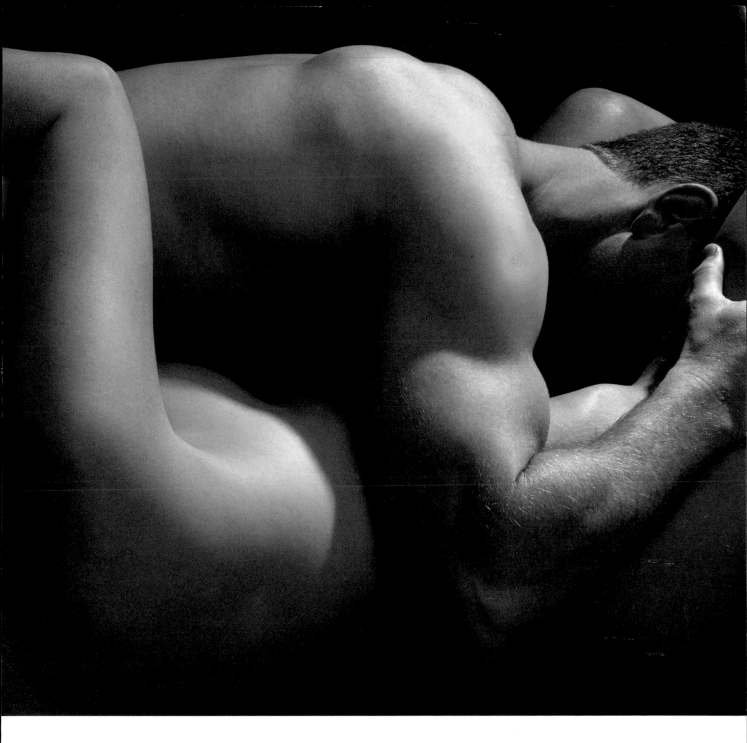

tives, and ligament-straining positions worthy of the Kama Sutra.

2. Scenes of sexual irresistibility. Here the emphasis is on seductive power— overcoming the reluctance of an initially indifferent man through sheer animal magnetism. Or the irresistibility may take numerical form in fantasies involving multiple partners.

3. Dominance and submission fantasies. In these, sexual power is expressed ritualistically—in sadomasochistic activities— or through physical force, as in rape fantasies. Such fantasies are surprisingly common. Studies have found that 51 percent of women fantasize about being forced to have sex, while a third imagine, "I'm a slave who must obey a man's every wish."

Coming Attractions

Here is a sampling of fantasies women
have shared.

"I'm sleeping naked and I wake up
to feel the tip of a tongue tracing slowly
down my forehead, over my nose, and over
my lips where it lingers. I open my eyes to
see a strong-jawed, well built man leaning
over me, watching me intently with a look of
lusty desire. I am shocked and a little fright-
ened, but then desire takes over. My mystery
man slowly lowers the covers to reveal my
breasts and he slowly continues exploring me
with his tongue, from my lips down my body
around my breasts, over my nipples, over my
stomach, and down to my wet pussy.

"He begins kissing my neck and then
sucking my nipples, softly at first and then
harder as his desire grows. I am the helpless
damsel under his power. He throws the covers off to completely expose me, lifts up my
knees and continues kissing me down my
body, on the insides of my thighs, and over
and around my clit. "After I come hard, he
pushes himself up against me and makes love
to me frantically until we both come and lay
there in a heap of covers and sweat. After
that he gets up and gets dressed and leaves
me lying there to go back to sleep."

"We are at a party and this beautiful woman
comes up to me, and says, 'I would like to go
home with you and your husband.' She
spends the weekend with us, dressed in
opaque silk, quiet, lovely to look at, with a
sharp mind and a glimmer of mischief in her
eyes. She gives us both deep and sensuous
kisses, smoldering glances, and we take her
to bed in turn and together.

"When she is dressing to go, I stop her,
remove her clothes, touch her between her
legs and make her whimper. My husband
watches us, aroused as we linger in the door-
way, I clothed, she naked. We ask her
to stay and she agrees to three more nights.
For those three days she is our seducer
and lover. My husband takes her from behind
in front of a mirror while I masturbate; she
goes down on me while he watches, stroking
himself. Every night she slips into our room,
her hair loose, her nipples so erect and red-
dened we know she is aroused and longing to
be taken. On the last night she slips away to
her room and beckons one of us and then
the other to pursue her and play out her
desires and ours.

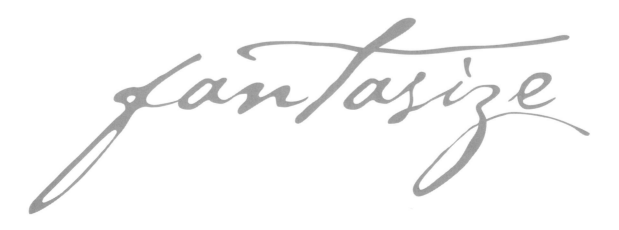

fantasize

"I fantasize about having mad, raw, no-guilt sex with my husband's law partner. We are in the parking lot of their office building. He kisses me first, I tell him "no," but I kiss back. He pushes me into the back of his truck and I rip his clothes off. He lifts my skirt, turns my back to him, and has his way with me. Every time I think about it I nearly have an orgasm."

"I have a fantasy that I go to my psychiatrist for some advice about my dirty thoughts. As I am telling him my thoughts he is becoming very aroused and he gradually moves his chair, which is on rollers, closer to me. He winds up sitting very close, and he has these really intense dark eyes that I find compelling. He leans into me and asks if I would be willing to open my mind to a powerful solution he has. The word 'powerful' resonates with me, especially because he looks at me very intently with those dark, mysterious eyes when he says it.

"I nod and feel myself getting very aroused. He tells me that I'm a naughty girl and that the only way I will get over my impure thoughts is to act them out once and for all. As he is telling me this, he slips his hand up my skirt and he says that as my shrink it is his job to help me. He drops his pants and he is very hard and very big. He pushes me onto his couch and I explode with excitement as he enters me. It is only after we're done, while I'm gathering my belongings, that I glance over at a coffee table and spot a textbook that he wrote on sex therapy."

Some fantasies may be soft and romantic, others may involve sex out on the edge with a stranger, and still others may be violent, sadomasochistic, or involve same-sex partners, sex with multiple partners, or sex in a public setting. Studies conducted in the past decade have shown that men and women's fantasies are becoming more alike, with women reporting more graphic and sexually aggressive fantasies than they had in the past.

Should you worry about your fantasies? Probably not. In fact, there may be more need to worry if you don't fantasize! Fantasies drive arousal, facilitate orgasm by blocking out worries and concerns, and allow us to explore taboo but hot activities without taking any risks.

It is emphatically clear: Your brain is a vital part of the sexual experience. Mental distraction can spark conflicting, nonsexual impulses in the brain and lessen your pleasure. In contrast, mental pictures of you on Hump Island surrounded by delicious sex partners drive your libido.

Bottom line: Vivid and sustained fantasizing is not optional; it is the second step in speeding up orgasm.

Studies on easily orgasmic women (those who climax more than 90 percent of the time) have found they anticipate steamy encounters for hours, even days. Indeed, fantasy's power to arouse—some women say they can achieve orgasm solely from sexual thoughts, or "thinking off"—proves that the brain is as potent a sexual organ as one's genitalia.

Though most erotic thoughts are relatively ordinary, our more imaginative flights allow us to explore our sexuality without risk of physical harm or social rejection. Consider this finding: Imagining having sex with your current lover is a popular fantasy when you're not engaged in sexual activity, while imagining sex with a new partner is a popular fantasy during intercourse.

People who are more physically active have more sex, better orgasms, and richer fantasy lives than non-aerobic exercisers.

FANTASY 101

Priming your brain for sex isn't always intuitive. For example, you probably think watching the woman of the hour cuddle onscreen with her latest hunk of the hour will put you in the mood, but you might be better off renting the latest action flick to kick your body's sympathetic nervous system into high gear.

For a long time most of us thought we had to be relaxed to get in the mood. However, current research suggests that raising heart rate, breathing, and muscle activity just before sex enhance your body's ability to get turned on. So if you're not an athlete, watch a movie to amp things up. As your body revs up and becomes aroused, turn to your guy and give him that hungry look.

More brain food can be found in your local bookstore. Read erotica. Women tend to think about sex less than men. But the more you think about sex, the more attractive it becomes. It's a simple technique, but very powerful. Not comfortable walking up to the counter at your local bookstore with a handful of dicey books? Browse in private by doing an online search for erotica on popular bookseller Web sites.

Yes, exercise feeds the brain and the results filter down between your legs. You don't have to train like you're an Olympic hopeful, just get more active. People who are more physically active have more sex, better orgasms, and richer fantasy lives than non-aerobic exercisers. Physical activity may increase natural testosterone levels (which fuels desire in women as well as men), and it helps pump blood down to erogenous zones, like the vagina, increasing sensation. Regular activity also boosts your energy, improves your confidence in your appearance, and confers a sense of general well being, all of which can give your libido a lift.

It is also essential that you believe in your sex appeal. If you are obsessing about how lousy you look, chances are your libido is going to head south. Stand in front of a full-length mirror naked for a few minutes a couple of times a week and eventually you'll see something you appreciate—your smooth skin, the shape of your breasts, or your luxurious hair. Whenever you walk by a mirror, practice seeing those sexy parts (instead of focusing on what you *don't* like about your body). Doing so will reinforce a more positive, sexier body image.

Sometimes, putting off the pressure to achieve orgasm can be wonderfully freeing and erotic. It's a technique pulled from my fellow sex therapists' bag of tricks: deliberately hold off from intercourse or orgasm for days or even weeks while exploring more subtle erogenous zones on each other's bodies. Thinking about a hot encounter, putting it off, flirting, and teasing creates the kind of tension that begs for release. Over the course of a few days, build to increasingly more erotic caressing and eventually to sex. In the meantime, you'll accumulate a series of positive and intimate sexual experiences that will make you want to go back for more.

You can also condition yourself to have an orgasm with no hands—almost. Using the bridge technique during intercourse, your guy (or you) stops the direct clitoral stimulation just at the point of climax so you can concentrate on the sensation of his strokes as you orgasm. Each time you have intercourse, stop stimulating your clitoris a bit sooner; if you do this gradually, you will have created a mental trigger for your orgasm.

FAIRY TALES THAT COME TRUE

Think about sexual fantasies as the cornerstone of your sex life. Whatever shape your fantasies take, exploring them can open doors to understanding your arousal and can allow you to tap into new channels of erotic expression—channels that work for *you*. Think about your fantasies whether they are vivid, vague, or a little scary.

Don't try to look too deeply into your fantasy's meaning; keep your mind open, and don't pass judgment on yourself—it's not about good or bad, it's about letting your mind roam free. To make use of your fantasies, to make them a driving force that heats up your sex life, try the following suggestions:

1. Write six scenarios each. Be as wildly imaginative as you like but limit the actors to the two of you.
2. Together, pick from the lists something that both of you find exciting. Don't pressure your partner to try something he or she finds distasteful, embarrassing, or uncomfortable.
3. Adapt the scenario for the real world and go for it.

Tip: Whatever the fantasy, whether in your head or acted out, look into your guy's eyes at the moment of orgasm. The image of your lover in the throes of pleasure is an incredible turn-on for most women.

1. Think about how comfortable your partner will be discussing this type of sexual activity. Some people might find violent, aggressive fantasies disturbing. Some might respond unfavorably to hearing that their partner fantasizes about group sex. There's nothing wrong with pushing each other's comfort levels; in fact, it is often beneficial, but doing so takes care.

2. Preface your sharing with some general discussion of fantasies, what they mean and don't mean. You might want to read some of my earlier remarks out loud to your partner.

3. Be reassuring about your partner's desirability. Some fantasies may make your partner jealous. For example, he may feel threatened by hearing that you fantasize making love to someone else, particularly someone else who's hot.

tion first," a thirty-six-year-old woman reported. "It never went past flirting, but then we would go home and role-play the scenario. It pumped up the erotic tension and made for hot sex, but never crossed the line into reality. We always left the bar together, just us!"

5. Let your partner know there's no pressure to act upon the shared fantasies. You both may decide it would be fun to try fantasy acting, but sharing shouldn't turn into coercing.

6. Remember that sharing is a reciprocal activity. The other person has a right to say, "I don't find this erotic at all." Be receptive to your partner's fantasies, too. You aren't the only one with a secret inner life.

QUICKIE
BATHS AND SHOWERS

"I'm exhausted, I could really use a good soak," you tell him when you get home from work. You kiss him lightly and go into the bathroom, where you turn on the taps and strip off your clothes, pour in some bath oil and step into the warm, rushing water.

The door opens and he comes in. "Mind if I join you?" he asks. He leans over the edge of the tub to kiss you and you latch on, throwing an arm around his neck and pulling him toward you. His blue denim work shirt is soaked when he leans away. "Hey!"

You splash water at him, completely soaking him. In mock anger, he strips off his clothes, and you pretend to be shocked as he dives for you. The water sloshes on the floor and you turn off the faucets so that you can dunk each other.

He pours shampoo into his palm and massages the bubbles into your hair. Then he lets his soapy palms move down your neck and shoulders, and makes circles of bubbles around your breasts. He lets his other hand roam further down so he can stroke your pubic hair.

You pour some more oil into your palm and starting with his thighs, you move up and stroke around his testicles and back between his legs. You tease him, decorating the tip of his erect penis with soap, gently dusting it off, and then applying the soap more vigorously.

He pulls you to your feet, releasing the catch so that the water starts to drain. "Got to get all this soap off," he says, turning on the shower. He adjusts the nozzle so that three powerful streams of water issue forth, and he holds you so that your back is flush against his chest, the water directed to your breasts, your belly, and your vulva. He tells you to spread your legs and you do so, allowing the water to

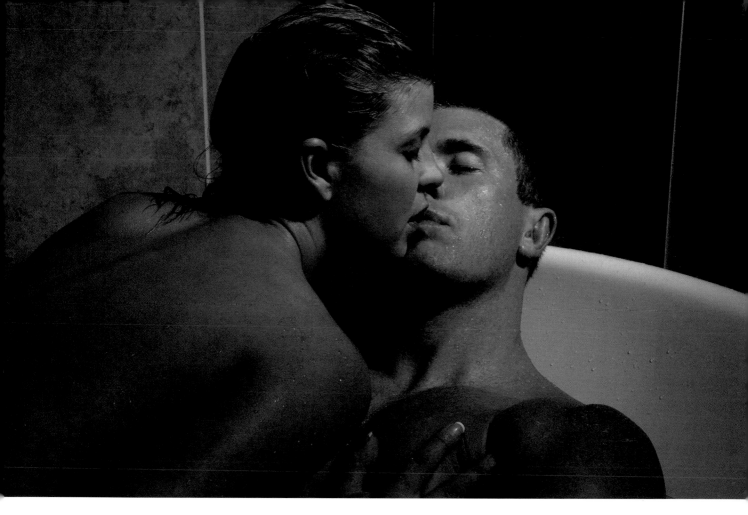

spurt up into you, creating a wave of such
pleasure that you buckle against him. He
turns the nozzle again, giving you a fine mist
that trickles between your buttocks.

arousal

You pull the sprayer out of his hand
and turn it on him, raising his arms to
wash between them, tickling his ribs, and
finally switching on one strong stream of
water and running it along the length of his
penis and up toward his ass.

You cling to each other as you step from
the tub wrapped in one big bath sheet, wrig-
gling together for a moment to get dry while
enjoying the sensation and building arousal of
skin on skin.

He cups one breast and you draw him
closer. The room is steamy, but not only
because of the hot water. Standing skin to skin,
he enters you gently and fully. You have just
as hot a time dry as you had wet, maybe
even better.

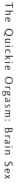

The Quickie Orgasm: Brain Sex

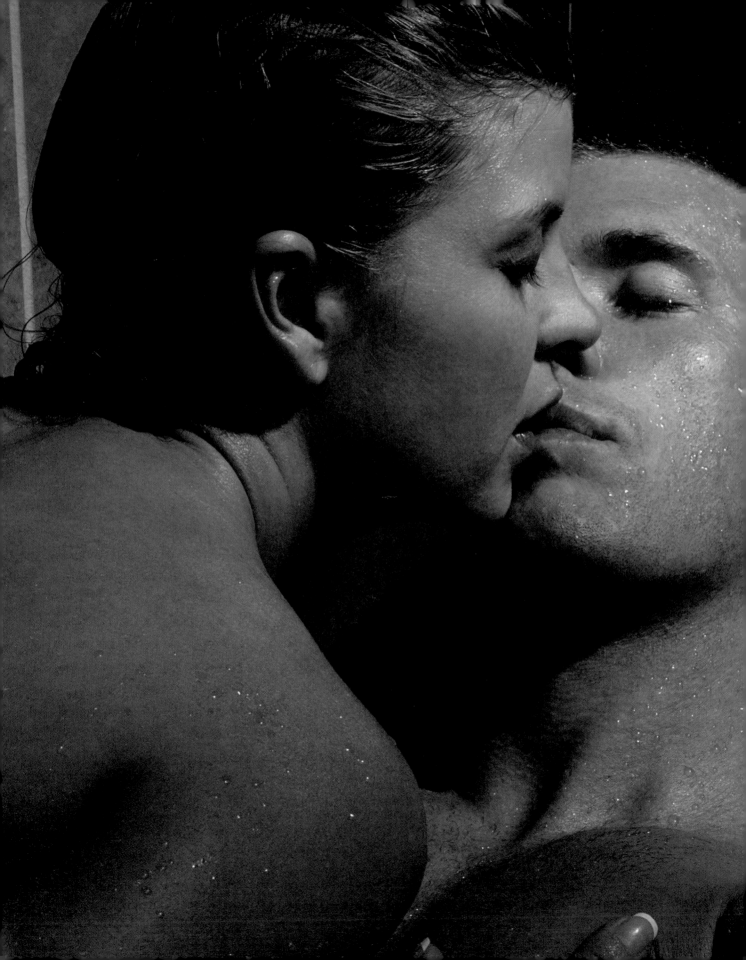

8

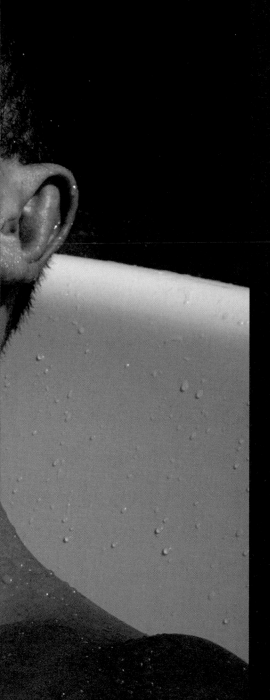

The Quickie Orgasm: Get in Position

A Woman's Place is on Top

Sex is like dancing. There are millions of moves, and most of them are unnecessary. Like dancing, there is no right or wrong, it's all about those few moves that make you feel good. In other words, when it comes to intercourse, it's about positions that stimulate the spots that get you over the top, especially the C-spot.

With the right partner at the right time and place, great sex involves friction and fiction. Fiction is the movie you show in your head; friction is the boost you give your orgasm through direct stimulation of your hot spot.

We've seen that reaching orgasm is not simply a lucky shot in the dark. If you want your juices to flow and you want it now, thinking sexy and positioning yourself for maximum friction in just the right spot is necessary.

To stimulate your C-spot during a quickie or just plain vanilla sex, it is essential that you take charge. Quickie sex and faster orgasm is about being bold. Some women who experience orgasm during intercourse unconsciously attempt to bring the focus to the clitoral area for maximum contact. If you're one of these women, that's excellent. If you're not, it is important you make an intentional effort to position yourself so that you get the clitoral stimulation you need.

This is the way men get stimulation as well, but it's easier for them. By moving the penis against the vaginal wall, they are receiving the kind of stimulation they need during intercourse—you should be doing the same thing, directing the stimulation to where it feels good.

FIRESIDE

WHEN THE WOMAN IS ON TOP, SHE CAN CONTROL THE DEPTH OF PENETRATION AND THE PACE OF THRUSTING, WHILE THE MAN CAN BE VISUALLY STIMULATED BY WATCHING HER PLEASURE HERSELF AND RHYTHMICALLY MOVE.

Granted, quickie sex in locations other than bed may not always lend itself to ideal positions. Hopefully the compromise will be compensated by the excitement of the moment. However, for fast orgasm, whenever you can, climb into girl-on-top position, arch your body toward him and grind your pleasure point against his pelvis.

The key to satisfaction is steady stimulation in a position that hits your pleasure points. You need to develop a rhythm, and once you feel yourself building toward climax, keep the sensation consistent so that you continue the momentum.

There isn't anything magical about you being on top, but it does have one big advantage—it gives you control of the action, and ultimately, greater freedom of movement.

Ride 'em

When you are on top, you control the depth of penetration and the pace of thrusting. You manipulate the amount of friction and the speed. You have the ability to shift slightly from side to side, or more brazenly you can bend forward with your breasts touching his chest, even sliding your breasts back and forth, stimulating your nipples against his chest. And, of course, you are able to reach down and stimulate yourself directly.

To give you another source of erotic pleasure, you can also lean back with your hands supporting you behind your shoulders, your clitoris pressed firmly against his pelvic bone. Some women, in the final moments of intercourse prior to orgasm, flatten themselves out on top of their guy, clench their thighs together and roll their clitoris into him.

Another move that may help is to grind your hips horizontally instead of (or in addition to) moving up and down. This will give your guy the same friction and sensation while simultaneously grinding your clit into his hips, which may very likely boost you into orgasmic bliss.

One of the other benefits of being on top is that your guy gets to watch you enjoy and pleasure yourself with your body. He gets to watch as you reach orgasmic heights while your hands are free to rub, hold, scratch, and maneuver your body. Talking to guys confirms this—they say it is the most visually stimulating position because they can admire your breasts and see your face when you reach orgasm.

A sizzling spin of you-on-top involves lowering yourself onto his penis in a kneeling position. Keeping your knees on the bed, hook your feet over the inside of his legs, likely at his knees. Grab the bed sheets on either side of his head, squeeze your butt, tilt your pelvis upward and move in small, tight motions.

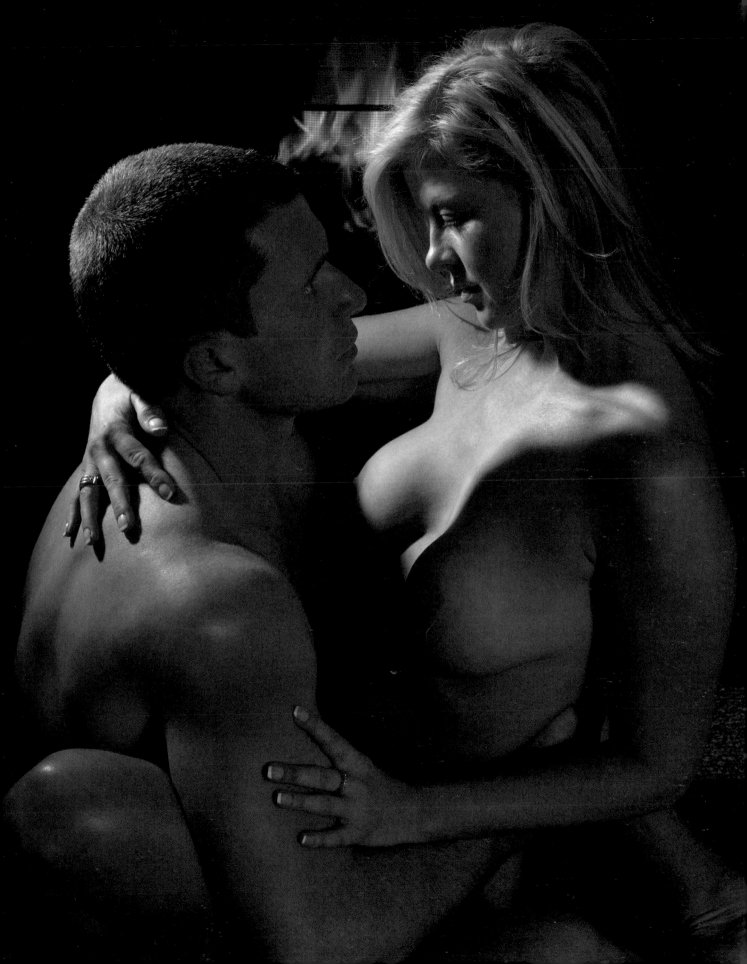

By gripping the bed sheets and using his legs as stirrups, this quasi-cowgirl configuration offers lots of leverage, so you maintain a steady rhythm without losing momentum before reaching orgasm. And since your body is higher than it is typically, your clitoris can rub against his pubic bone.

Yet another variation involves your guy lying on his back, then sliding down the bed until only his upper back and head are supported, with his feet on the floor supporting his weight. Standing, you straddle him, and use your legs to thrust up and down. The advantage for you is that you have complete control of the angle, speed, and depth of the thrusts, and you also have freedom of movement because you're supporting your own weight. His hands are free to stimulate you wherever you like—and so are yours. Keep your legs braced during your orgasm, as your knees might go wobbly for a while.

One more sizzling variation of you-on-top is to have your guy lie back with one leg outstretched and the other bent, so his knee is pointing upward. You may call this a thigh-master, but this is one that actually works!

Facing sideways, lower yourself onto his penis and hold on to his bent knee for leverage. As you rock back and forth, lean far enough forward so your joy button rubs against his inner thigh. This torrid two-in-one move makes you the center of amorous attention: the steady thrusting plus constant clitoral contact against his inner thigh will prime you for a big O. And with his leg right there to balance you, you're free to really let go and grind in wild motions.

There are numerous other variations, some of which should be reserved for couples that have a background in gymnastics. The point is that standard intercourse is an inefficient way of reaching orgasm. For a faster orgasmic response, it must be supplemented with a position that lends itself to direct clitoral stimulation, usually involving either his hand or yours.

With you on top you get more bang for your buck! You are afforded clitoral stimulation while having the freedom to shift during intercourse and the ability to easily reach down and provide additional stimulation.

Here's what a forty-something woman had to say about her experience.

"This is a great position for a woman who knows how to excite a man. My sex life has improved tremendously since I learned how to make the best use of it. I make eye contact with my husband, especially when I come. My husband told me that his first wife always closed her eyes when she came. He felt cheated because she hid her vulnerability from him. I use my hands. Guys get very aroused watching a woman touch herself during intercourse. And, I'm a little dominant when I'm on top. I lean over and tweak his nipples occasionally. Or take his wrists and push them over his head."

Bottom line: Step three of your three-phase program toward faster orgasm is to position yourself for direct clitoral stimulation during intercourse. This is crucial for your success.

If you have body image anxiety that stops you from getting on top and your guy's reassurance isn't enough to alleviate your concerns, you

sizzling

can wear a short silk robe, a nightie, or any sexy piece of lingerie that makes you feel more appealing. You don't have to be completely nude to make love. Clothes can give you confidence, even in bed.

HE RIDES YOU—
DIFFERENTLY

Maybe you simply favor the position with him on top. You're not alone. Here's what one forty-seven-year-old woman said.

"I like the missionary position best because we can go at it better in that position than others. I move my legs from his shoulders to around his waist. Sometimes I plant my feet on either side of him. I can thrust harder in that position. Sometimes I lie absolutely flat. It feels different each way."

The missionary position is actually the most popular for intercourse, but for most women it will not provide the needed clitoral stimulation. It's sort of an engineering problem—a man's thrusting simply does not apply enough friction to the clitoris.

It would be like you rubbing his testicles. You're off the mark, but if you do it long enough, you may just coincidentally create some friction closer to where it needs to be—the head of his penis. For some men, close may be good enough, but for most, it's not.

The same applies to women. Most women need more direct clitoral stimulation than comes with the missionary position, especially if they want to speed up their response. It's all about clitoral stimulation. To get the best stimulation you need to take charge. Being on top puts you in charge of the firmness, rhythm, and pace of the clitoral stimulation. Especially if you have been masturbating, you are the world's expert on your own sensations and it makes sense for you to provide the sensations. Being on top allows you to do so easily.

Having said that, some women still are more comfortable in the bottom position. All is not lost. Being comfortable, both physically and emotionally is important.

Here are four simple variations of guy on top that will up your odds for ecstasy.

1. The coital alignment technique (also known as the CAT). Your lover climbs on top, but instead of entering you in the usual "missionary" way, he lies so that his pubic bone is actually rubbing against your clitoris. By settling into a gentle rocking rhythm, his penis rubs against your clitoris while he's moving in and out of your vagina.

   In the CAT your lover's body weight is on you—but what if he is built like a SUV? You can also get clitoral stimulation when he raises his body and rests his weight on his elbows or his outstretched arms.

2. He places his legs outside of yours, while you keep yours together. This placement increases the friction.

3. Raise your legs so that your knees are pressed to your chest and your legs are draped over his shoulders. This will give you more friction and pressure exactly where you need it—your vaginal lips and clitoris.

4. Sit in a chair or on the edge of a low bed, thus allowing your guy to kneel on the floor for thrusting. For heavyset men it can reduce the weight he places on you, and allows for both of you to reach your genitals. The downside is that some women consider this position to be less intimate.

Once again, these position suggestions may not always be possible during quickies. It depends on the circumstance and location. But since your sex life is not going to one quickie after another, being in a position that speeds up your orgasmic response whenever you can is not a bad thing. In fact, it's a very good thing!

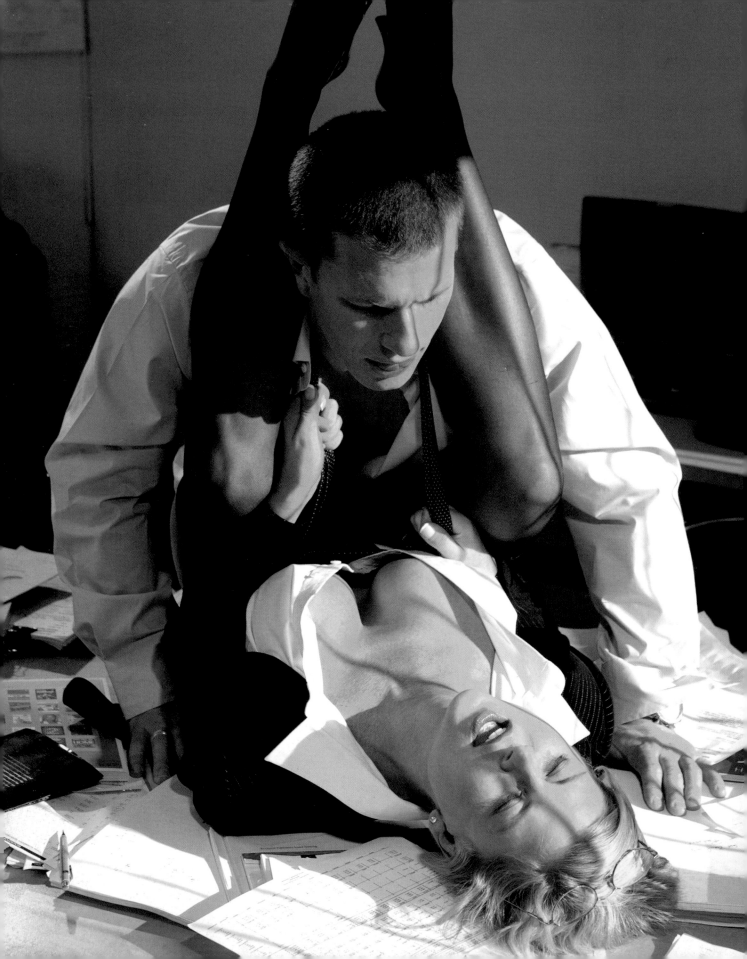

MID-MORNING COFFEE BREAK

WHO SAYS YOU CAN'T MIX BUSINESS WITH PLEASURE? IF YOU DO TAKE A MID-MORNING QUICKIE "COFFEE BREAK," MAKE SURE YOUR OFFICE DOOR IS LOCKED AND THE SHADES ARE DOWN SO YOUR COWORKERS DON'T CATCH YOU IN THE ACT.

IT'S YOUR BODY—TAKE CHARGE

You may already realize that some of the phenomena happening to your body during sex are under your control. While you cannot voluntarily increase and decrease your heart rate, you can take charge of various voluntary activities and thereby improve your sexual sensations. Consider the following powerful tips:

1. As you approach orgasm, try speeding up your breathing and alternately tensing and relaxing your arm or leg muscles.
2. During another session of lovemaking, practice squeezing or fluttering your PC muscles.
3. Have an active orgasm by bearing down during intercourse, pushing the same muscles you would if you were trying to dispel something from your vagina—this helps you push down against his penis and the result is a longer and more intense orgasm. (It'll make his penis pay attention as well!)
4. The main behavioral principle is to choose one physical aspect of orgasm that you can control and over-practice it. Soon you will train your body so that all of these responses work together effortlessly and occur spontaneously during future orgasms.

To get the best stimulation you need to take charge. Being on top puts you in charge of the firmness, rhythm, and pace of the clitoral stimulation.

QUICKIE
LUNCHTIME INTERLUDE

You call him at the office in the morning. "Sweetheart," you say, "check your briefcase—I left something in there for you." Inside he finds a sealed envelope on which you've written, "Guess what's for lunch?" Inside the envelope is a pair of edible panties.

The exciting thing about this time together is that it's got to be quick, so you suggest what you'd like to do to him on the back of the envelope. "All I want for lunch is you," paints an explicit picture, as does "You make my mouth water."

When he walks through the door, you're not there. Instead, he hears the sound of music coming from somewhere else in the house. You've taped a piece of paper to the banister. A red arrow piercing a heart points in the right direction.

You wait behind a door (not necessarily the bedroom door) with only your underwear on and a bunch of grapes in your hand. You put on a favorite CD, and the shade on the skylight is raised, letting sunlight stream over your body.

You undress him. Don't let him lift a finger to help while you punctuate your movements with little teasing endearments—a kiss in the hollow of his neck as you rip off his tie and then his shirt; a soft stroke on the inside of his thigh as you undo his belt buckle, pop the button, and pull down his zipper. You cup his penis and testicles with both your hands and tell him how warm he is and how hot you are.

You let the clothes fall away and quickly drape them over a chair (remember, he has to get back to the office after this). You start in a standing position, holding one another and exploring the territories that are usually hidden in the dark. See where the sun hits you and direct his kisses to those places—under your arm, behind your knee, at the nape of your neck. Wrap one leg around him so that he can easily reach under the elastic of your panties.

Now snake out of your panties and expose yourself to him completely, letting him see all of you. Let the sun caress the curve of your breast, the roundness of your belly. Put his hands just where you want them as you run the tip of your tongue around his lips. Take a grape into your mouth and gently, as you kiss him, transfer it to his. Put a cluster over his penis and suck on each one until you reach the flesh.

When neither of you can stay on your feet because of your excitement, drop to your knees and put your arm around his neck. He is fully erect so you move forward and straddle him, moving slowly back and forth, gripping him with your thighs.

He has a committee meeting at two, and you have a project to finish by the end of the workday. So this is the time. You take the lead, pushing him onto his back so that you can be on top. Together, you polish off that lunch and more.

QUICKIE

WELCOME HOME

A LUNCHTIME QUICKIE IS A GREAT WAY TO FEEL A LITTLE NAUGHTY, ESPECIALLY WHEN YOU'VE RETURNED TO WORK AND YOUR LOVER'S SCENT IS STILL FRESH ON YOU. DURING THAT BORING AFTERNOON MEETING YOU CAN DAYDREAM OF YOUR HOT LUNCHTIME ESCAPADE.

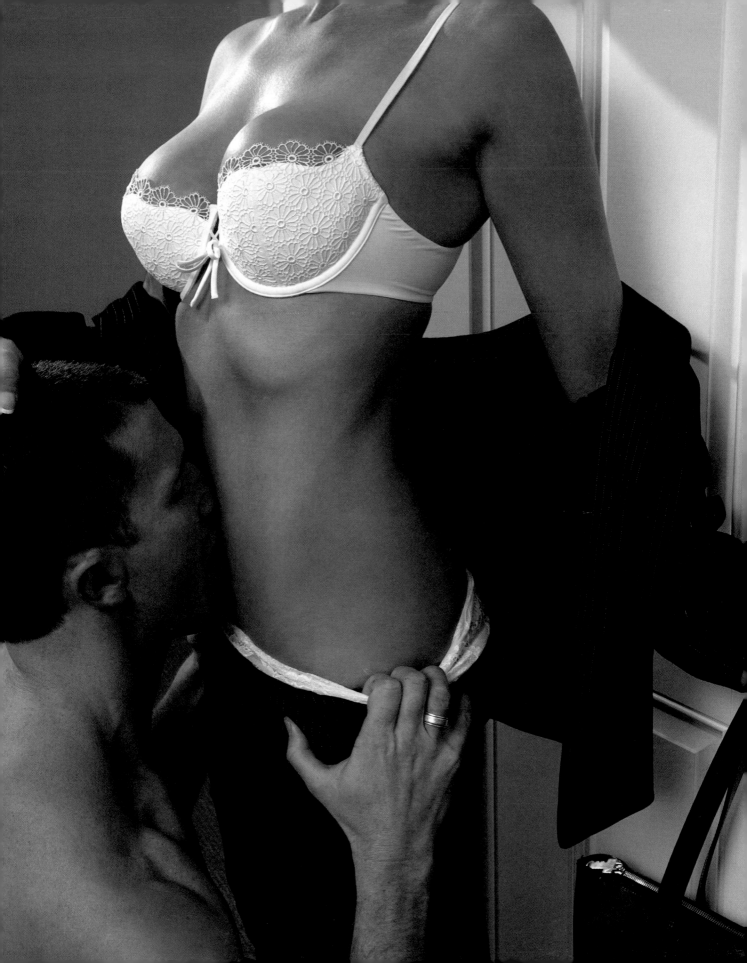

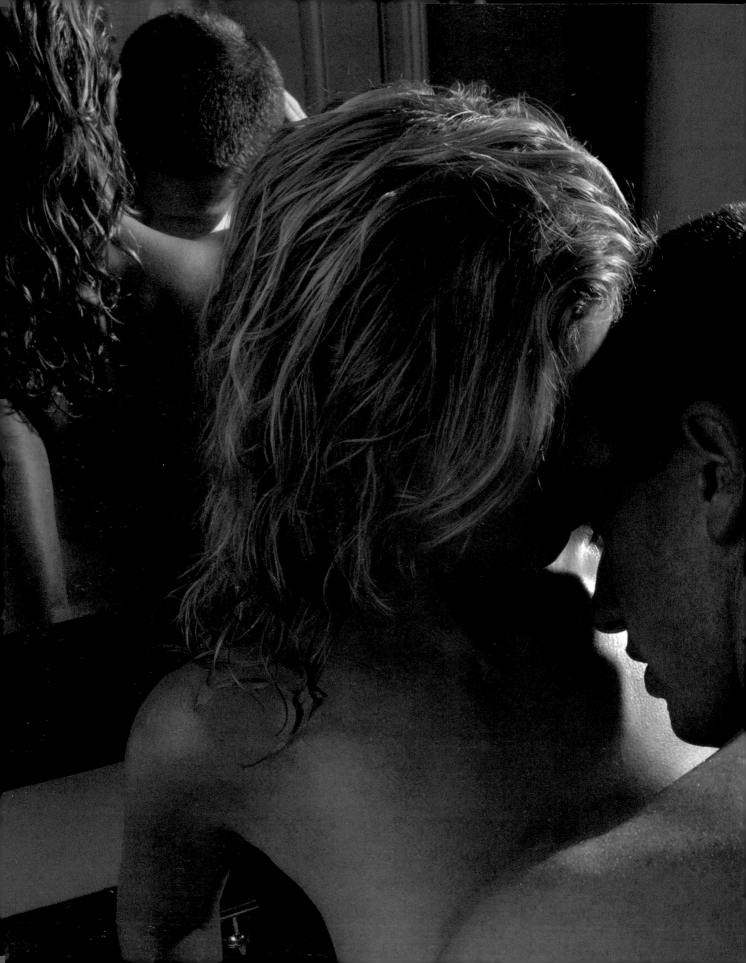

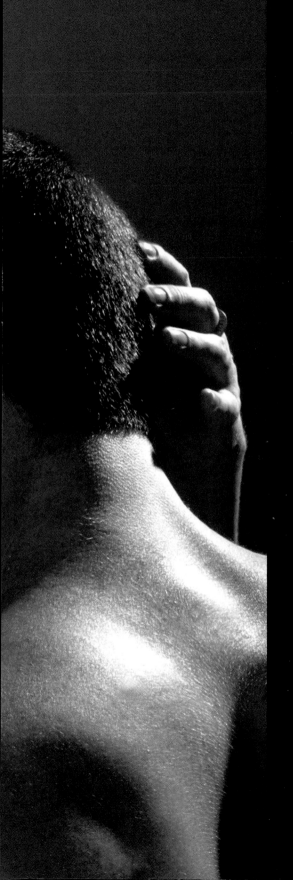

9
Putting it All Together: The Orgasm Express

Some easily orgasmic women simply may be physiologically fortunate. They may have a clitoris that is either larger than average or positioned so that the shaft of the penis effortlessly strokes the clitoral region during intercourse. But if you are not one of those fortunate women, there is still a lot you can do to quicken and intensify your orgasms

1. **Pleasure yourself.** You are comfortable with masturbation and pleasure yourself regularly. Masturbation encourages greater sexual awareness. There is no better way than masturbation to know and understand your sexual response and how you react to definite physical stimuli. It is the best training for quickening your orgasmic response and essential for catching up with your partner during sex. And don't forget to stimulate yourself, using your wise and experienced finger, during quick sex.

2. **Talk dirty.** You aren't embarrassed to ask for what you need or to stroke yourself during lovemaking. More to the point, you feel entitled to your pleasure and will ask your partner to use his hand, or you will use your own hand or a vibrator to stimulate your clitoris during intercourse. You are also comfortable letting him give you a "head" start with a one-minute visit downtown. (Remember, studies show that oral sex has the double bonus of quickly lubricating and stimulating you in all the right places.)

3. **Position yourself.** You've learned how to align your body with your partner's body and move your hips so that you get the kind of clitoral stimulation you need. Anything that presses down on your lower abdomen during intercourse—his hand or your hand—is likely to create more clitoral contact. In addition, clenching your buttocks and your upper thigh muscles will increase blood flow to your entire pelvic area. Increased blood flow leads to greater vaginal lubrication and clitoral engorgement, which pushes nerve receptors closer to the surface for greater sensation.

4. **Breathe fast.** In the heat of passion, thinking about breathing may be the last thing on your mind, but intentionally quickening your breath pattern can help increase an orgasm's impact—the faster you breathe, the more excitement you're likely to experience. Breathing through your nose may be good for reducing stress, but in matters of the big O, breathing through your mouth is where it's at.

Thinking about breathing may be the last thing on your mind, but intentionally quickening your breath pattern can increase an orgasm's impact.

5. **Think impure thoughts.** Freely entertain thoughts and fantasies rather than trying to suppress them out of guilt as some women do. Screen out sex-negative messages. A study in the *Archives of Sexual Behavior* revealed that women are very stimulated by erotic images (although your body's response may take a while to catch up with what's going on in your brain), so keep the lights on and your eyes wide open. You may even want to move that mirror into position for a closer look.

6. **Stay positive.** Avoid attitudes that inhibit orgasm. These include the following:
   > He's tired, or I'm taking too long… I'll hurry up.
   > He should give me an orgasm.
   > I shouldn't have to tell him what I like.
   > Pleasing him is more important than pleasing myself.

7. **Think hot sex.** Do this and it's more likely to happen. Okay, sex isn't going to cure you of those nasty habits you've been agonizing over all your life and it is not going to influence world peace. But, even if it feels as though you're just going through the motions at first, stay hot with anticipation for what's to come (you!) and your body becomes more responsive very quickly.

8. **Avoid speed busters.** If you want to go from zero to sixty in less time than it takes you to finish with your makeup in the morning, here's some behavior to avoid:

    > Not kissing first. The lips are not only hot, but letting him dive straight for the erogenous zones may give you a pay-by-the-hour feeling. That can be a bummer—unless, of course, that's exactly what you're looking for.

    > Breaking contact. Maybe the quickie isn't always the most intimate coupling, but unless you are intentionally looking to make it feel like anonymous sex, keep in physical contact with each other. Stroke each other, rub your bodies together, or lean into each other, but stay physically connected. It makes a difference in how you feel about the experience, which makes a difference in how you will respond.

9. **Drink up.** Drink lots of water and skip the toilet break before sex. Research suggests the many woman experience powerful orgasms as a result of the increased abdominal pressure of a full bladder.

10. **Go easy on the lube.** Commercial jellies have gotten so good that, for some women, they're too good—overcorrecting to the point of eliminating too much friction. Try saliva or water instead.

THREE PHASES TO FASTER ORGASM

Reducing the steps to a bare minimum— the three-phase program for faster orgasm:

1. Masturbate to prime your sexual responsiveness and become an expert on the touch that turns you on.
2. Make love with the improper stranger— fantasize.
3. Position yourself so that you are able to provide direct clitoral stimulation during intercourse.

Bonus Time: The Extragenital Orgasm—and More!

I'm going to throw in some challenges here that you may not be able to achieve, but if you don't permit yourself to feel frustrated, the experiences will enhance your pleasure even if they don't result in orgasm.

The point is to have some techniques on hand that increase pleasure and deepen sensation. You will be cheating yourself if you use them to set orgasm goals or if you measure your performance against the women commenting here, or anywhere on these pages for that matter. We'll discuss the extragenital orgasm first, then the spontaneous orgasm, and lastly the simultaneous orgasm technique.

The Extragenital Orgasm

An orgasm achieved with no genital contact is an extragenital orgasm. Relatively few women report being orgasmic simply from kissing passionately or by having their nipples kissed, their thighs caressed or licked, or other parts of their bodies nuzzled. How can it be done?

Women who experience extragenital orgasms are able to excite themselves through erotic thoughts and fantasies to the point where any form of physical stimulation sends them over the edge into orgasm.

If you want to try experiencing one, follow these suggestions:

> Have a more traditional orgasm first. Some women can experience an extragenital orgasm more readily after they've had an orgasm through clitoral stimulation. Be sure to show a sexy movie in your head throughout the experience. The fantasy for this experience better be very hot, perhaps a daring quickie you've had, or one that you've thought about that very much excites you.

> Caress or have your partner caress your genitals until you are on the verge of orgasm. Switch the stimulation to a nongenital area such as your breasts or thighs.

> Alternate from genital to nongenital stimuli until you are so close to orgasm that a simple touch like running a finger down the inner thigh could induce it.

Here's what a forty-four year old woman said about her experience:

"The orgasm occurred in an alley behind a bar filled with my friends celebrating a birthday. He was by himself having a drink and our eyes met. Not a word was exchanged. He simply motioned toward the door and I slipped out of the bar as if I was in some kind of lustful trance. The next thing I knew my arms were pressed to the wall behind me and he kissed me with the most incredible passion.

"He didn't put his hand up my shirt or down my pants, but an orgasm just burst from me. All the while my friends were in the bar on the other side of the wall I was up against; any one of them could have could have wandered out in search for me. I think the secrecy made the encounter feel more illicit, which added to the excitement, even though I wasn't cheating.

"We saw each other for a few months after that. He was twelve years younger and talked about having a baby. I knew it was dead-end, but it was charged and sexy. It finally fizzled out because it was too much trouble to keep it secret. My friends would have written him off as 'Mr. Wrong,' and I never even told him about my twenty-two-year-old twin daughters!"

The Spontaneous Orgasm

If the nongenital orgasm sounds like a challenge, how about a spontaneous orgasm, the ultimate no-hands solitary sex experience? The spontaneous orgasm occurs with no physical stimulation at all. According to limited research on the subject, a few women can actually think themselves to orgasm. One researcher not only interviewed women who claimed to have this experience but measured their physical responses in a clinical setting and proved their claims had merit. How do they do it?

> Set the atmosphere. Take a bath, have a glass of wine, put on some music, dim the lights.

> Create a lush, passionate, and emotional sexual fantasy. Really move into it.

> Lying on your back, knees bent, feet spaced well apart, take deep breaths. Pull your breath into your body so deeply you can feel your diaphragm expanding and can imagine air going all the way down to your genitals. When you breathe out, pull that air all the way out, again imagining you are drawing it up through your genitals into your body.

> Pant. After a dozen or so deep breaths, pant. Breathe rapidly from your belly with your mouth open.

> Flex the PC muscles either alone or in combination with the breathing. Coordinate your flexing with deep breathing. Switch to panting, then back to deep breathing—all the while flexing PC muscles.

> If you don't have an orgasm this way, don't despair. Most women won't. But use the technique during masturbation or intercourse and see how much stronger your orgasm is.

A thirty-eight-year-old woman reported this experience with spontaneous orgasm:

"I am easily orgasmic, capable of multiple and extended orgasms, but I couldn't make this one work. I could get to the point where just touching my clitoris a few times brought me to orgasm. However, I recommend the exercise, simply because it leads to an incredibly intense orgasm when you finally give up and touch yourself."

Touch

The Simultaneous Orgasm Technique

Some couples still believe that the ultimate expression of sexual intimacy is the simultaneous orgasm. In films and novels that were popular in years past, the lovers almost always appeared to come at the same time. Their ecstasy at the same moment left little room for alternative interpretations. Women—the consumers of more romantic fiction—particularly believed mutual climaxes were better than separate but equal ones.

In fact, the simultaneous orgasm is more serendipitous than typical. The belief that they should climax when their partners did led some women to fake an orgasm at the propitious moment, and then feel secretly angry and dissatisfied afterward.

In real life, men typically reach orgasm before women do, and women are far more capable of multiple orgasms than men are. However, I am betting that if you have been with me thus far, you are becoming more easily orgasmic and you are more closely aligned with the timing of your partner.

Despite your growing advantage, simultaneous orgasm shouldn't be the ideal. Some couples like to experience it occasionally because they enjoy the special intimacy that coming together brings to lovemaking. With a little attention to timing and advance planning, you can make this technique work.

> Time your response cycles so that you know approximately how long it takes for you and your partner to reach orgasm during your most typical lovemaking pattern.
> Assuming it takes you longer than it does him, let him stimulate you alone until you reach the point where you are the same distance away from climax as he will be when stimulations begin for him.
> Communicate with each other. If one of you is moving faster toward climax than anticipated, say, "Slow down."

Weighing in on the experience of simultaneous orgasm, a forty-two-year-old woman, married for ten years, had this to say:

"My husband, in contrast to other men I've been with, is good at timing himself and waiting for me. I'm sure some people just coincidentally come together, but we mostly manage it by knowing each other well enough to balance doing good things to each other and making sure good things get done to ourselves.

"It works best for me during intercourse. Somehow I've never managed simultaneous orgasms during mutual oral sex. I find I get too distracted focusing on him to concentrate on my own sensations, which may be lack of practice. It requires less coherent effort for me to keep up the simpler and mostly instinctual hip action involved in plain old screwing. But I will say this: I think coming together is neat. It adds to the already weird moment of distorted consciousness at the peak of orgasm, because we are both in that state at the same time."

A Note on Pressure versus Pleasure

We are a very competitive society. As a consequence, this discussion of "super" orgasms and the discussion we are going to get into in the following pages—seriously super orgasms, called multiples—can make you feel like you have to reach the pinnacle of erotic bliss or else you're a failure. That's a mistake.

Orgasms are joyous events, regardless of how they occur and how they are experienced—sometimes they are more intense and sometimes a mere blip on the blast-off screen. If you pressure yourself to have an orgasm that is a rocket ride to another dimension, you are destined for disappointment.

The maxim here is enjoy the process and the orgasm will be there for you—forcing it, or demanding some sort of super orgasm will doom you to failure.

THREE TIPS TO AMP UP YOUR ATTITUDE

1. **BECOME MORE SELF-INDULGENT.** When people have a lot of responsibilities they begin to feel guilty about taking any kind of pleasure, from a long hot bath to an afternoon at the movies. This attitude is certain to affect sexuality. Luxuriate in small pleasures.

2. **LEARN HOW TO STOP NEGATIVE THOUGHTS.** When you can't stop thinking about the irritations and injustices of the day, make yourself stop. Each time you have a negative thought, hit the pause button on the mental VCR. Replace it with a positive thought.

3. **GIVE EACH OTHER PERMISSION TO BE SOMEONE ELSE.** Have you become trapped in your roles—parent, jobholder, caretaker of aging parents, and so on? Play like children. Pretend for the night that you are characters from a favorite book or film or even fairy tale. A new role may set your libido free.

pleasure

QUICKIE
THE LOVE GAME

You arrange to meet at a bar and agree that you will pretend not to know each other. The one who arrives second has to play the pick-up artist. When you arrive he's waiting in the lobby bar of an upscale hotel. The ambiance is elegant. A long, highly polished mahogany bar is flanked by a mirrored and richly carved back bar. The drinks are expensive and the clientele look well off. You take the bar stool one over from his and he pretends to ignore you, affecting an expression of world-weary ennui so well worn by the rich and celebrated.

Though you don't smoke, you pull a cigarette from your tiny handbag and pretend to search for a light before turning to him and murmuring, "I can't find a match. Do you have one?"

"No one smokes anymore," he says, half turning away from you. In response, you make a half turn toward him, uncross and cross your legs and look at him with a bemused expression on your face until he can't resist looking back at you.

"I was quite sure you were aware of me," you say, pitching your voice seductively low.

"It would be hard to miss those legs," he says.

"Are you a leg man?" you ask. You put your hand on one knee and slowly move it up your thigh, exposing a little more leg encased in sheer black stocking. Lowering your head and raising your eyes, you look at him from beneath the broad brim of a stylish black hat.

"I can be," he says, deliberately not meeting your eyes, but keeping his gaze on your leg.

"I'll bet you can," you say. "Are you staying in town long?"

"I live here," he says, turning to face you now, his leg brushing yours. "And you?"

"I'm here to collect an inheritance," you say. "A former lover died, and left me with a bundle. Grateful, I guess."

SEX ON THE COUCH

SEX ON A SOFA CAN BE EXCEL-LENT, PARTICULARLY BECAUSE OF THE GOOD SUPPORT IT GIVES YOU FOR A VARIETY OF DIFFERENT POSITIONS.

He raises his eyebrow and grins. That was creative and quick. He puts his hand on top of yours, the hand that is still resting on your thigh.

"Let me buy you a drink," he says. You know you have him.

An hour later, you're groping each other passionately in his car parked in the hotel garage. You're going to "his" place. You are, you say, a little drunk and ready to toss your virtue aside.

"I like it hard and hot," he whispers in your ear. "How about you?"

For an answer, you take his hand that was covering your breast and squeeze his fingers until they compress your nipple tightly. A shiver runs up your spine. He roughly pushes aside the fabric of your V-necked dress, reaches inside your black-lace bra, and finds your nipple. As he thrusts his tongue deeply into your mouth, he twists your nipple and you moan appreciatively.

Before he starts the car and begins the drive home, he shoves your skirt up, exposing your genitals. You're wearing a garter belt and stockings, no panties. At every stoplight, he inserts a finger into your vagina. By the time he pulls into the garage at "his" apartment, you're wet.

Inside the apartment, with a panoramic view of the city before him, he takes you the way, he says, "A man takes an expensive slut": from behind as you are bent over the sofa. Your orgasm is both profound and prolonged. He deliberately stops himself from coming because, he knows, after both of you have changed clothes and driven back to the hotel to get your car, you will make love again, playfully and maybe more tenderly this time.

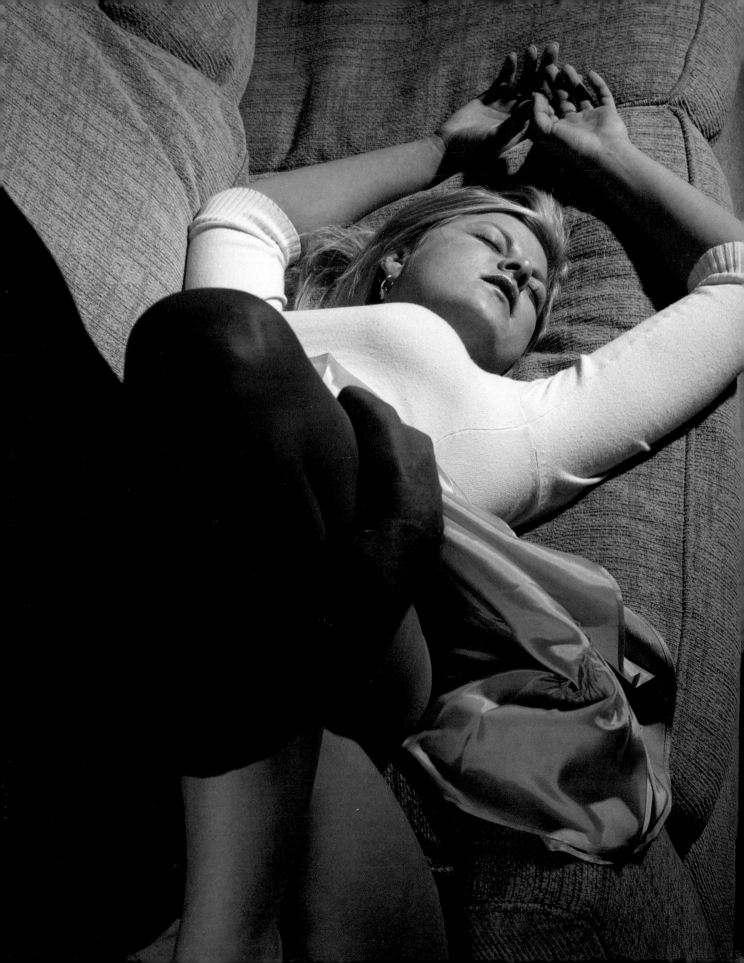

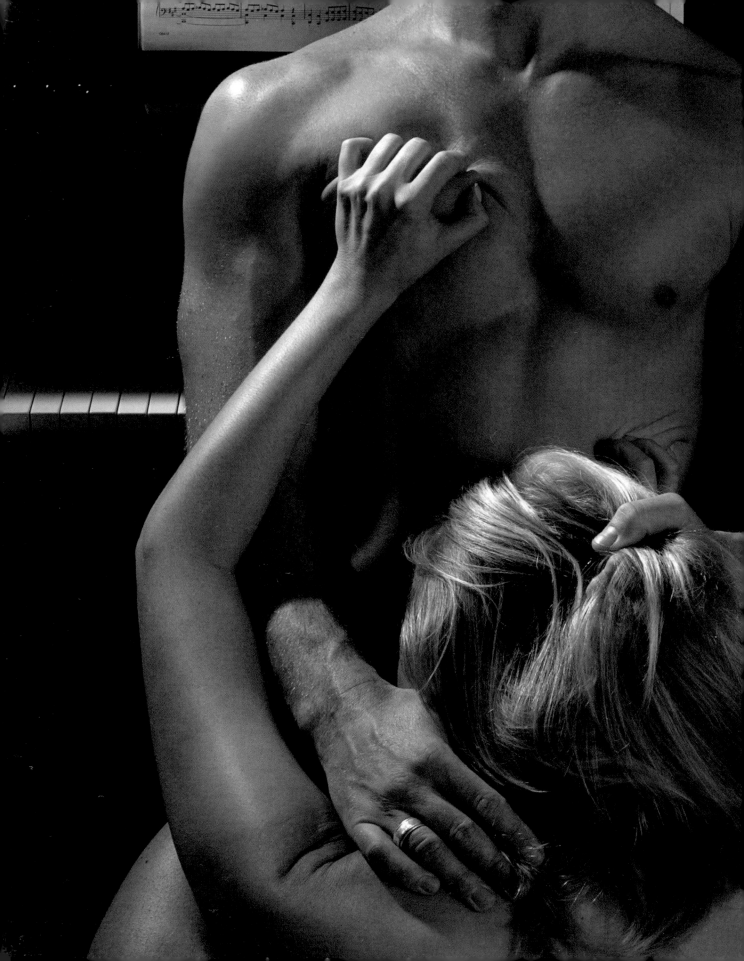

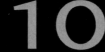

10

Going for the Gold: Multiple Orgasms

YES, YOU CAN!

We've gone through the extragenital orgasm, the spontaneous orgasm, and the simultaneous orgasm. Now what? Multiple orgasms during a quickie? Okay, we may be pushing it, but don't rule it out! There may not be a lot of time, but when you bust out of the usual routine and turn the heat way up, you never know what will happen. Besides, if you've been bringing a smile to his face with sex at unexpected times in unexpected places, he will surely be pleased to help you have more than one orgasm, even if it's in the rush of the moment.

Let's begin with what "multiples" are—orgasms that occur when you have a second or third orgasm or more without completely returning to the resolution phase (the "I'm done moment"). In other words, a level of excitement is maintained between orgasms; you are not starting the climb up again from a low point on the arousal scale. Most women are capable of having multiple orgasms though it may take some practice—and practice must work because women are definitely getting better at it!

In the 1940s, the American sex researcher Alfred Kinsey found that one in seven women experienced multiple orgasms. Another researcher found the figures to be much the same. However, in the 1960s, Masters and Johnson discovered that, given enough stimulation, most women were capable of having more than one orgasm. They found that, in most cases, a woman was "capable of having a second, third, fourth or even fifth and sixth orgasm before she was fully satisfied." Many of the women were able to have five or six full orgasms within as many minutes.

A more recent survey of 106,000 American women of all ages showed that 67 percent usually have multiple orgasms, with one in seven of those over thirty-five years old saying they have multiple orgasms every time they make love. Of those who had multiple orgasms, 66 percent experienced between six and ten orgasms, and 6 percent experienced eleven or more.

After practicing the three-step program I've described in previous chapters and revving up your sexual engine with quickie sex, you are now more likely to have multiple orgasms. Once you've put yourself in an accelerated sexual mode, your erotic responses are more rapid, your level of confidence is higher, and your sexual awareness is greater.

It's been my experience that for many women, regular orgasms or multiple orgasms begin to happen now because they've finally gotten over the embarrassment of needing manual clitoral stimulation during intercourse to achieve orgasm. They've also sexualized their lives through fantasy—with anticipation of the next quickie! Indeed, once you feel free to touch yourself or ask for the touch, and you give yourself permission to watch a dirty movie in your head, you not only quicken your orgasmic response but you also notch up your chance for a multiple.

Still not a believer? Eight hundred and five nurses can't be that wrong! In a study reported in the *Archives of Sexual Behavior,* these nurses answered a detailed questionnaire about sexuality and all stated having multiples

orgasms. It was found that women with multiple orgasms don't just get them by accident. Having identified what they like, they choose the techniques that maximize their pleasure and communicate to their partners what arouses them most.

The study found that women who have multiple orgasms are definitely different in how they approach their sexuality. They are more likely than those who don't experience multiples to examine their clitoris, and to both give and receive oral-genital stimulation. They like their bare breasts fondled and their nipples kissed. They are more likely to enhance clitoral stimulation during intercourse by thigh pressure or masturbation. Multiple orgasmic women are also more likely to engage in mental stimulation via erotic fantasies, films, and literature. These are precisely the factors that we've been discussing and you've been practicing!

There are several different types of multiples, including the following:

> **COMPOUNDED SINGLES.** Each orgasm is distinct and separated by a partial return to the resolution phase.

> **SEQUENTIAL MULTIPLES.** Orgasms occur two to ten minutes apart with minimal reduction in arousal between them.

> **SERIAL MULTIPLES.** Mere seconds or minutes separate numerous orgasms with no diminishment of arousal. Some women experience this as one long orgasm with spasms of varying intensity.

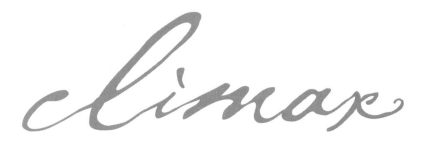

THE TECHNIQUES

Mental attitude, as always, is key. First, if you haven't discarded the idea that lovemaking ends with your guy's ejaculation, do so now. His orgasm isn't the signal for the end of lovemaking.

Next, you need to focus on your own pleasure to achieve multiple orgasms. Shut out intrusive thoughts and prepare for multiples by fantasizing about sex before the encounter, teasing yourself mentally and caressing your genitals in the bath or shower. Having a glass of wine isn't a bad idea either, unless you have a problem with alcohol.

Once you're in the right frame of mind, here are the five most powerful techniques:

1. **ALTERNATING STIMULI.** For some women it's not only the right kind of stimulation that counts, but the right kind of *varied* stimulation that makes the difference.

Ask your partner to give you the first orgasm via cunnilingus. Oral sex more fully arouses the female genitalia, making orgasm during intercourse more likely.

After the first orgasm, he should manually stroke you to yet another orgasm if possible.

If you do not reach orgasm easily by manual stimulation, revert to oral.

After a second orgasm, have your guy immediately enter you, with either of you continuing manual stimulation at the same time. Some women report that intercourse at that point seems to "spread" the sensations of orgasm throughout the body.

Maintain a pattern of varied stimulation as long as desired. Once you've climaxed, simply change your lovemaking position—or even shift within the position—and get a slightly different type of stimulation.

After you've climaxed, your vagina will tighten and then contract. If your guy alternates between stroking the inside of your vagina and your clitoris, you'll keep on feeling the contractions every few seconds until you're completely taken over by an involuntary full-face smile.

Here's what a thirty-four-year-old woman who experienced multiple orgasm for the first time had to say:

"Alternating stimuli, with the first orgasm via cunnilingus, works for me. Other methods haven't. In fact, I like two oral orgasms. After that, if I'm in the right mental place, I can fly. I feel myself soaring into a level of pleasure I'd never reached any other way."

2. **MANUAL CONTACT.** Women who aren't comfortable touching themselves during lovemaking are less likely to experience multiples because they have to depend on their partners to know exactly where and how to apply the stimulation that will take them from one peak to the next. Even the best lovers can't always get it right, so it is important that you become comfortable with this first.

> Stroke yourself during cunnilingus or intercourse.
> Vary the stimulation to the clitoral area.
> When you feel orgasm approaching, move the stimulus from the clitoris to the area surrounding it to spread the orgasm.

A forty-something woman reports: "I can have multiple orgasms in a variety of ways. I'm one of the lucky women. Manual stimulation is the surest way for me to get there. From masturbating, I know exactly when, where, and how to touch myself to bring on the spasms. My husband is an excellent lover but he can't pinpoint the site and pressure changes that take me from one orgasm to another as fast as I can. Besides, he loves it when I touch myself."

3. **REPEATED DIRECT STIMULI.** While some women are more likely to have multiple orgasms using alternating stimuli, others have a better chance of doing so if their partner repeatedly stimulates the clitoral area in the same way. These women need constant, concerted stimulation at the focal point to have multiple orgasms. The beauty of the clitoris is that it's like the Energizer bunny that keeps going and going, not needing R&R after climax. For these women, as long as the stimulation continues, the orgasms keep on coming. Many women, however, find the clitoris too sensitive to sustain this pattern of stimulation.

For women who are put off by this because of their sensitivity, the secret is to use other methods of indirect clitoris stimulation. Caress the entire vulva area (staying away from the clitoris), perform regular intercourse, or stimulate some other part of your body altogether.

One woman, twenty-something, talked about favoring the "stay with it" technique: "I can keep having orgasms if I or my partner continues stimulating my clitoris throughout and beyond the first orgasm. Sometimes the clitoral area gets so sensitive, I think I can't bear the touch. If I don't pull away, the acute sensitivity passes. I move into a place where I sometimes feel like I could come forever."

4. **THE FLAME.** Some women have multiple orgasms only during cunnilingus. This technique, which should be used in addition to the other suggestions above, often works. These directions are for your guy:

> Pretend the tip of your tongue is a candle flame.

> In your mind's eye, see the flame flickering in the wind.

> As the candle flame moves, move your tongue rapidly around the sides, above, and below her clitoris.

Comments from a woman turning fifty years old: "This is nirvana. I don't know where my husband learned it. He said he got it from a book. Wherever he picked it up, I'm glad he did. After the second or third orgasm this way, my whole body feels like it is convulsing. I'd never had multiples until he pulled this trick out of his bag."

5. **G-SPOT MULTIPLES.** Some women have multiples only when they receive both clitoral and vaginal stimulation in the area of the G-spot. Again, these directions are for your guy:

With your palm facing her, insert your lubricated index finger and middle finger into her vagina. Push gently around the outer third of her vagina's top region until you find the sensitive place, a rougher patch than the surrounding skin. Make a "come, hither" gesture, stroking her G-spot.

FINAL TIPS

Getting to the point where you experience multiple orgasms takes some practice, but once you've learned to be more easily orgasmic, it's easier to have multiples because your genitals are already engorged and your body is awash with the potent chemicals of sex. It may take a few minutes to reach the first summit, but once you're there, the rest of the climb is faster and you're likely to soar with the joy of it. Here are some final tips.

ADDING POWER TO THE EXPERIENCE: FOUR TIPS FOR SUCCESS

1. **THINK MULTIPLE.** You are more likely to have multiple orgasms when you visualize yourself having the experience.

2. **BREATHE THROUGH YOUR CLIMAX.** When you feel yourself close to orgasm, inhale, then try to time your exhale with the onset of the orgasm. You'll feel the sexual charge flow through your body to your toes.

3. **START EXPERIMENTING DURING MASTURBATION.** Next time you feel especially sexy, perhaps around period time, get very aroused and then, when you have had one orgasm, experiment with other ways of stimulating yourself until you have another. If you usually climax with your fingers stimulating your clitoris, try a vibrator around the area until you come again.

4. **ADORE YOUR GENITALS.** A new study, led by women's health expert Dr. Laura Berman of Chicago's Berman Center, shows that there are statistically significant positive relationships between a woman's genital self-image and her sexual satisfaction. Women with a higher genital self-image also show higher sexual function and have a higher quality of life, according to the study.

breathe

Or, during intercourse in a position that is favorable for G-spot stimulation, such as the rear-entry position, stroke her clitoris.

Individual differences and response patterns vary so much that no woman should feel pressured to find her G-spot and then reach orgasm this way. Reaction to stimulation in the G-spot region varies greatly among women. Some are sensitive, others are overly sensitive, while still others report little sensitivity at all. Consider these far ranging comments:

From a thirty-year-old woman: "I can't find my G-spot if I have one. I've explored, my boyfriend's felt all around the area. We've both searched. Nothing! I don't think I have sensitivity there."

From a thirty-five-year-old woman: "I think I have found the spot, or rather my boyfriend has. It gives me pleasure when he strokes it, but nothing extraordinary. The G-spot is not the next clitoris. Sometimes it takes me a while to feel what he's doing with the G. But when he strokes my clitoris, I know!"

ORAL SEX TUTORIAL

FELLATIO IS ALWAYS A WELCOME WAY TO SATISFY A MAN.

From a woman in her forties: "This works for me, especially in the rear-entry position where I get the best G-spot stimulation. One reason the position works is that I stimulate my clitoris. I still like to have the first orgasm via cunnilingus, and then switch to rear-entry intercourse and manual clitoral stimulation."

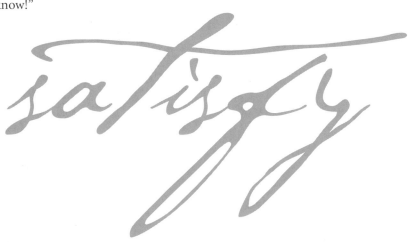

satisfy

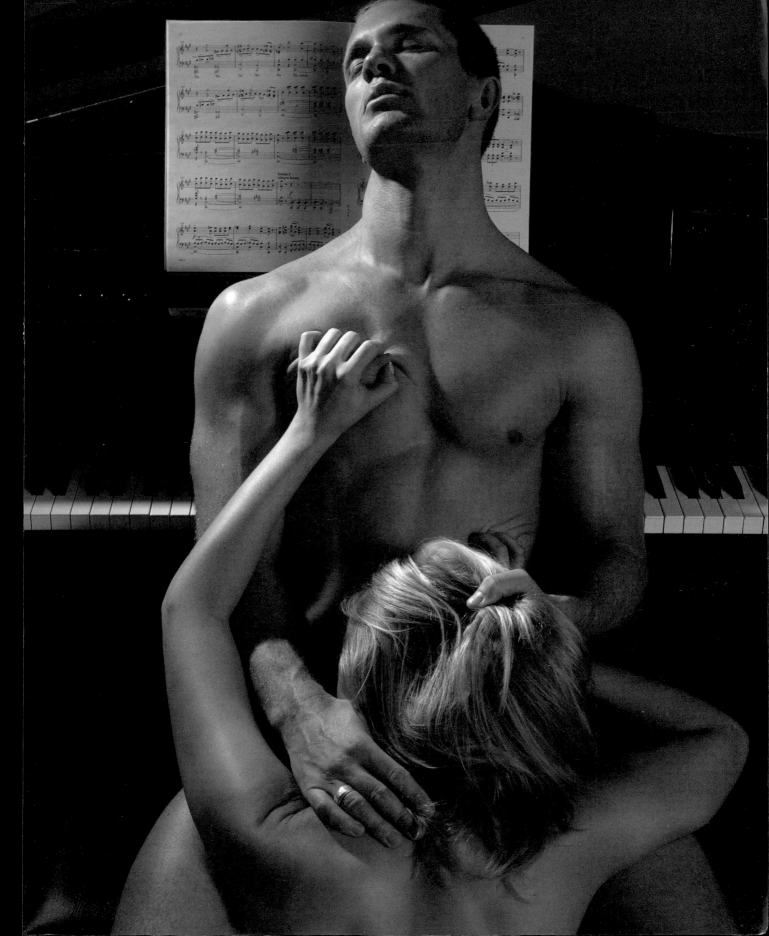

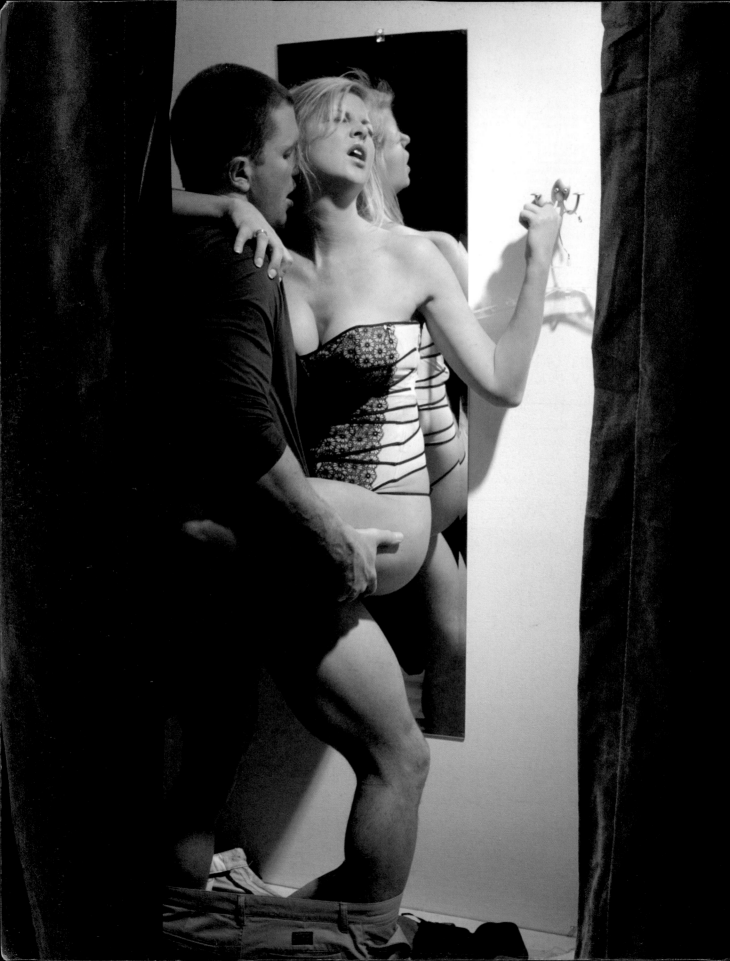

Sources for Erotic Videos, Toys, and Books

What's Out There?

Ah, so many toys and so little time. Variety can be both a blessing and a curse. It's nice to have options, especially sexual options, and it's super cool to have options when it comes to sex toys and erotica.

Your naughty desires may not be the same as another woman's, so it's good to have choice. But too many options can also be daunting, especially if you're new to the world of sex toys.

Let's start with a basic Sex Toys 101. First, by far the most popular sex toy for women is the vibrator. For some women a vibrator allows them to be more easily orgasmic, or allows them to have an orgasm during regular sex when they normally wouldn't. Many women have their first orgasm with a vibrator, and most women find it easier to reach orgasm with a vibrator than by any other way.

I strongly recommend vibrators that are meant to stimulate the clitoris; these are used externally, rather than being inserted into the vagina. Regardless of what you envision when you hear the word "vibrator," the external kind is the most effective for having orgasms and the most commonly used by satisfied customers.

If you buy a vibrator that uses an electrical outlet rather than batteries, the Society for Human Sexuality recommends the Hitachi Magic Wand. They state that in comparison to other plug-in models, the Hitachi Magic Wand is easier to use during sex with a partner, easier to put a condom over in case someone else wants to use it, and the optional penetrative attachments are of higher quality.

Of course, taking an outlet-based vibrator on the road for quickies isn't going to work, so pick up a battery-powered vibrator as well. The smallest of them can easily be kept in a purse and you can use it more discreetly and spontaneously. Battery-powered vibrators are also more convenient for partner sex, especially if you and your partner like to change positions a lot—no one will get strangled in the cord! Some of them can even be used in or near water (think "beach").

The Society for Human Sexuality recommends The Waterdancer as the most versatile choice. It's very small, very well made, and completely waterproof, with a design similar to that of the famed (but non-waterproof) Pocket Rocket.

What do users say about their experience with a vibrator?

From a thirty-six-year-old woman: "The vibrator is the easiest way for me to have an orgasm. I love it when my husband does it to me because his technique is better than mine. We sit on the floor or on the bed, my back to him, with him snug up against me. Lots of skin contact! He reaches around with one arm and uses the vibrator on my clitoris while holding and stroking me with the other hand. He also keeps a vibrator in the glove compartment in the car; you never know when we might need it!"

From a thirty-one-year-old woman: "My fiancé and I got a box of sex toys as a shower gift from friends. At first we laughed at the stuff. Then we decided to try it. We put honey dust on each other and licked it off, fastened each other to the bed with Velcro restraints and used the vibrator—with every attachment. Everything was very hot, but the vibrator, Wow!"

And from a forty-year-old woman: "When I was younger, I was embarrassed by the idea of using a vibrator with my partner. Now I enjoy using one with him occasionally, especially if we are going to have sex that is fast and furious. I like the idea of inviting my vibrating friend into the action, and he welcomes the extra help."

Your naughty desires may not be the same as another woman's, so it's good to have choices. But too many options can also be daunting, especially if you're new to the world of sex toys.

Sex Toys Tips

1. Make sure you have spare batteries. You don't want to be in the bathroom stall of your favorite restaurant and run out of juice.

2. When you're masturbating or having sex with a partner, do you prefer direct or indirect stimulation? Mild or strong? Focused on a specific spot, or spread over a wider area? Knowing what kind of play your body likes without sex toys is a good way to figure out what it might like when you do haul out the toy bag. If a vibrator is too intense for your bare clit, you can use it through panties, sheets, or a thin towel. Also, experiment with using the vibrator around your clitoris, not directly on it. The area surrounding your C-spot is also nerve-dense and will welcome the stimulation.

3. If you want to go for multiple clitoral orgasms, back off on the pressure after the first orgasm but keep the vibrator moving. Avoid direct contact with your clit until your arousal level builds again. Moving your hips while using your vibrator, perhaps also squeezing and relaxing your PC muscle in time with your breathing, may also enhance the experience.

4. If you're really clever you may be able to place the vibrator around your C-spot in a couple of different positions during intercourse, but you'll likely find that doggy style is the most convenient position in which to use the vibrator.

More Fun Toys

Once you've become comfortable using a vibrator on your clitoris, there are two other toys it might be fun to explore: a G-spot toy or a dildo. The G-spot toy is used to apply firm pressure against your G-spot, while a dildo allows you to enjoy a fuller and more satisfied feeling while using your vibrator. Not every woman finds stimulation of this area of their vagina to be enjoyable, but those that do really do.

Once again, the G-spot is an area on the forward wall of the vagina, about two to three inches in (just beyond the pubic bone). Particularly when you're very aroused, the skin may feel different from the area around it.

As I mentioned earlier, one way to stimulate your G-spot is by inserting a finger inside you, pressing firmly upwards, and stroking the area with a slight "come to me" motion. The other way to find and stimulate your G-spot is with a rigid curved toy.

If you use a Hitachi Magic Wand, pick up the Gee Whiz attachment for it. If you own a clitoral vibrator other than the Hitachi Magic Wand, the Society for Human Sexuality recommends the Archer Wand toy instead. This is also the best choice if you already know you like extremely firm G-spot pressure, or are having trouble finding your G-spot. If you don't own a vibrator but know you definitely want something that can stimulate your G-spot as well as your clit, the Society suggests the Nubby G.

Although G-spot stimulation isn't something that's enjoyable for every woman, women who do enjoy it will benefit from the use of these toys. By stimulating your G-spot as you approach and go through your clitoral orgasm, these vibrators will help you deepen and intensify your orgasms. Or, you may enjoy the G-spot stimulation as a sensation and source of orgasmic release completely on its own.

Sex Toys Tips II

1. Keep in mind that any toy you penetrate yourself with is going to feel better if you first apply a little water-based lube to it.
2. G-spot stimulation is likely to be hot once you're aroused, and the more aroused you are the hotter it may be.
3. Pressure may need to be quite firm and focused to get G-spot stimulation to work for you.

While G-spot toys are designed to intensely stimulate one particular part of the vagina, dildos are designed to give you a more generally satisfying feeling of fullness. When you have a clitoral orgasm with your vibrator, dildos can give you something firm and satisfying to clench your vaginal muscles around. They somewhat mimic the feelings experienced during intercourse with your partner, which may help you fantasize.

Your first choice in selecting a dildo is the material you want it to be made out of, and the best choice is silicone. Silicone is hypoallergenic and non-porous, meaning that you can either clean it with hot water and anti-bacterial soap, or completely sterilize it in boiling water for five minutes. It feels warm to the touch and retains body heat, transmits vibration beautifully, can be made into toys that range from floppy to almost completely rigid, and if taken care of (not exposed to anything sharp that could puncture or tear it, and not exposed to silicone lubes), your playmate could last a lifetime. In short, silicone is the perfect material out of which to make a dildo.

Your second choice when choosing a dildo is width and length, and the right width is by far the most important consideration because you can always adjust how far inside you insert the dildo. One way to pick a width is to use this rule of thumb: If you know that having two fingers in you feels just about right, select a dildo between an inch and an inch and a half in diameter. If three fingers feels better to you, pick something slightly larger than an inch and a half in diameter. If you'd like to be certain, first purchase some inexpensive non-silicone dildos in a variety of widths and try them out. Then choose the width of your silicone dildo based on which size felt the most comfortable to you.

The third choice you'll have to make is whether you want your dildo to resemble a human penis or for it to be less realistic looking. Those models that don't resemble a penis come in a variety of abstract textures and shapes.

Your final choice when choosing a dildo is the shape. Do you like the slightly eye-popping feeling of first being penetrated? Then pick something with a slightly pronounced head or knob at the tip. Do you like pressure against the forward wall of your vagina? Then pick something with a curve. In general, it's easiest to just look at the shape and imagine what it might feel like inside you and when entering you.

Yes, there are more sex toys that we could discuss, such as harnesses, anal toys (beads, butt plugs), bondage toys, and sex board games. But we're only presenting the basics here.

Shop Time

Sex is big business and you will find Web sites for sex toys all over the Internet. The list below is not meant to be exhaustive, but is a sampling of the reliable, well-run shops for sex toys, books, videos, and assorted erotica.

The following listings have a policy of protecting your privacy—they state that they do not sell customer information to third parties. Some well-known places to shop have not been included because, last I checked, it is their stated policy to sell customer information to third parties.

BLOWFISH

Mail-order catalog and Web site of toys, books, videos, DVDs, safer-sex supplies, S/M gear, comics, and magazines. They feature individual reviews of their products.
P.O. Box 411290
San Francisco, CA 94141
800 325 2569
415 252 4340
www.blowfish.com

BLUE DOOR

Buy or rent adult videos, with a nice selection divided into understandable sections. Videos are rated for excitement and entertainment and are individually reviewed by staff and customers
ETP, Inc.
P.O. Box 64378
Sunnyvale, CA 94089
724 772 6076
724 772 3048 (fax)
www.bluedoor.com

GOOD VIBRATIONS

Mail-order catalog, website, and retail stores carry toys, books, videos, DVDs, safer-sex products, magazines, and comics. All products are individually selected and reviewed. The vibrators have volume and intensity ratings, and the website is loaded with sex info and even a magazine. Mail order is open 7 a.m. to 8 p.m., PST.
938 Howard Street, Suite #101
San Francisco, CA 94103
800 289 8423
415 974 8989
www.goodvibes.com

TOYS IN BABELAND

Web site, retail stores, and catalog of toys, books, videos, and safer-sex supplies. Women-owned and operated.

Babeland New York—Lower East Side
94 Rivington St.
New York, NY 10002
212 375 1701
212 375 1706 (fax)

Babeland New York—Soho
43 Mercer Street
New York, NY 10013
212 966 2120
212 966 2144 (fax)

Babeland Los Angeles
7007 Melrose Avenue (near La Brea)
Los Angeles, CA 90038
323 634 9480
323 634 9481 (fax)

Babeland Seattle
07 E Pike Street
Seattle, WA 98122
206 328 2914
206 328 2994 (fax)

For online orders: 800 658 9119
www.babeland.com

Other Hot Books from Quiver

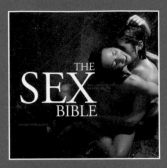

The Sex Bible
The Complete Guide to Sexual Love
By Susan Crain Bakos
ISBN-13: 978-1-59233-227-4
ISBN-10: 1-59233-227-7
$30.00/£19.99/$38.95 CAN
The Sex Bible is an authoritative, comprehensive, and beautifully pho-
tographed sex resource book that provides in-depth treatment of sexual
topics in frank detail. The book is arranged into different sections, including "Foreplay," "Sex Toys," and "Oral Sex." It explores sexual subjects you
are either familiar with, or until now, never even knew existed. Couples will
be captivated by personal anecdotes interspersed throughout. Illustrated
with full-color photography, *The Sex Bible* will not only educate couples,
but also it will help heighten sexual enjoyment.

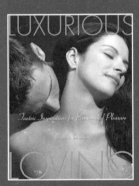

Luxurious Loving
Tantric Inspirations for Passion and Pleasure
By Barbara Carrellas
ISBN-13: 978-1-59233-237-3
ISBN-10: 1-59233-237-4
$19.99/£12.99/$25.95 CAN
Luxurious Loving teaches couples new, fun, and exiting ways to reincorporate
erotic and sensual techniques to their lovemaking sessions. Examining ancient
sexual practices and philosophies, such as Tantra and the Kama Sutra, as well as
modern sexual conventions, *Luxurious Loving* instructs readers on how to explore
each other's bodies through sensual head-to-toe touching, kissing, erotic massage, oral sex, masturbation, and numerous other playful turn-ons.

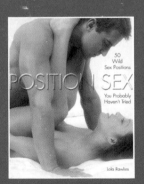

Position seX
50 Wild Sex Positions You Probably Haven't Tried
By Lola Rawlins
ISBN-13: 978-1-59233-238-0
ISBN-10: 1-59233-238-2
$19.99/£12.99/$25.95 CAN
For couples who might be stuck in a one-position nooky rut, *Position seX*
instructs couples on how to spice up their sex life and be more adventurous in
the bedroom (or any room, counter, or chair in the house.) The book features
full-color photographs of each hot, new position, as well as slight acrobatic
variations on good old standbys, such as the missionary position. In addition to
new positions, *Position seX* also provides tips on sexual accoutrements—dil-
does, vibrators, sexy lingerie, and lubricants—to further spice up your fun.